The Paramedic's
Guide to Research

The Paramedic's Guide to Research

An Introduction

Pauline Griffiths
Gail P. Mooney

Mc Graw Hill   Open University Press

Open University Press
McGraw-Hill Education
McGraw-Hill House
Shoppenhangers Road
Maidenhead
Berkshire
England
SL6 2QL

email: enquiries@openup.co.uk
world wide web: www.openup.co.uk

and Two Penn Plaza, New York, NY 10121-2289, USA

First published 2012

A catalogue record of this book is available from the British Library

ISBN-13: 978-0-33-524135-4pb) 978-0-33-524136-1 (hb)
ISBN-10: 0335241352 (pb) 0335241360 (hb)
e-ISBN: 978033541378

Library of Congress Cataloging-in-Publication Data
CIP data applied for

Typeset by Aptara
Printed in the UK by Bell and Bain Ltd, Glasgow.

Fictitious names of companies, products, people, characters and/or data that may
be used herein (in case studies or in examples) are not intended to represent any
real individual, company, product or event.

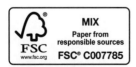

The McGraw·Hill Companies

Contents

6 Qualitative research in paramedic practice: an overview   73

Julia Williams

7 Using qualitative research methods in paramedic practice   90

Julia Williams

About the editors

Pauline Griffiths PhD, RN, MSc (Nursing), Post Graduate Certificate in Education, Post Graduate Diploma in Health Care Law is Senior Lecturer, Director of Pre-qualifying Studies, College of Human and Health Sciences, Swansea University, Wales.

Pauline has a clinical background in neuroscience and acute medicine. Her recent research interests include medical admissions units and the experiences of first-year paramedic students. Pauline has over 18 years experience in teaching research skills and providing thesis supervision and was the project manager for the development of the Paramedic Science Higher Education Pre-qualifying programme for Wales.

Gail P. Mooney MSc (Econ), FHEA, Post Graduate Diploma Social Research Methods, PG Cert Higher Education, RN is Director of Postgraduate Studies, College of Human and Health Science, Swansea University, Wales.

Gail's clinical background is in critical care having worked in a number of intensive care units. For a number of years Gail worked as a research officer and researcher involved in a range of research studies. She has been in education for the past ten years and has taught research methods and critiquing skills to undergraduate and postgraduate students. Gail led the curriculum team in the development of the All-Wales Diploma in Paramedic Science.

About the contributors

Jayne Cutter PhD, MSc, BN, DipN, RGN is a lecturer in the College of Human and Health Science, Swansea University, primarily teaching infection control but also research methods and statistics. Prior to this, Jayne worked for 20 years in the NHS in infection control, critical care and general surgery. Jayne takes the lead in teaching infection control to undergraduate paramedic students. She is also a member of the All-Wales Infection Control Policy development group.

Gary Rolfe PhD, MA, BSc, RMN, PGCert EA is Professor of Nursing in the College of Human and Health Science, Swansea University.

Gary's clinical background is in mental health and he has an academic background in philosophy and education. He teaches reflective practice and practice development and has published a number of books, book chapters and journal articles on philosophical aspects of practice, research methodologies, practice development and education. Since moving to Swansea University in 2003 he has worked with practitioners across West Wales to establish a number of practice development units.

Megan Rosser RGN, MSc Nursing Research, BSc Nursing, PG Cert Learning and Teaching is Director for Continuous Professional Development/Non-professional Undergraduate Programmes, College of Human and Health Science, Swansea University.

Megan has a clinical background in palliative care and oncology and lectures on pre- and post-registration healthcare related courses. Megan has a special interest in the application of research skills to promote evidence based practice.

Julia Williams PhD, PGCE, FHEA is Principal Lecturer and Research Lead for Paramedic Science at the University of Hertfordshire.

Julia has extensive experience both of undertaking healthcare research, and, since 1996, teaching research methods, and practice on degree programmes in Paramedic Science. Julia is an Adjunct Associate Professor at the Queensland University of Technology.

Malcolm Woollard MPH, MBA, MA(Ed), Dip IMC (RCSEd), PGCE, RN, MCPara, NFESC, FASI, FHEA, FACAP is Professor of Pre-hospital and Emergency Care at Coventry University, an honorary consultant paramedic, a registered nurse, an Adjunct Professor at Charles Sturt University and a Senior Research Fellow at Monash University, Australia.

Abbreviations

A&E	accident and emergency
APP	advanced paramedic practitioner
CAT	clinical assessment tool
CoP	College of Paramedics
CAQDAS	Computer Assisted Qualitative Data Analysis Software
ECP	emergency care practitioner
EMT	emergency medical technician
EBP	evidence based practice
DH	Department of Health
EMT	emergency medical technicians
GPs	general practitioners
HPC	Health Professions Council
INCD	Institute of Health and Care Delivery
IRAS	Integrated Research Application System
JRCALC	Joint Royal Colleges Ambulance Liaison Committee
LMA	laryngeal mask airway
MAU	medical assessment units
NHS	National Health Service
REC	Research Ethics Committee
NSF	National Service Frameworks
NICE	National Institute for Health and Clinical Excellence
NSF	National Service Framework
QAA	Quality Assurance Agency
PEP	post-exposure prophylaxis
RCT	randomised controlled trial
SIGN	Scottish Intercollegiate Guidelines Network

Research and the paramedic

Pauline Griffiths and Gail P. Mooney

Learning outcomes for the chapter
By the end of this chapter the reader should be able to:

1 Discuss the relevance of research to the practice and education of paramedics

2 Describe why paramedical practice can be classified as a professional occupation

3 Consider the development of paramedic education

4 Outline the basic stages of the research process

Keywords
changing role of the paramedic
paramedic education
profession

Introduction

The paramedic profession is at an exciting stage in its development. The origins of the profession lie in learning by rote and protocol controlled practice dictated by other professional groups. Ahead for the profession, if the challenge is taken, lies autonomous professional paramedic practice. To function at this level of responsibility and accountability paramedics need to be able to draw on research that has been evaluated critically to inform their *evidence based practice*. The College of Paramedics (CoP) (2008: 23) *Curriculum Guidance and Competence Framework* specifies that: 'The paramedic will be able to understand research *methodology* and clinical audit and be reading relevant research and discussing with colleagues the outcomes and conclusions'. Clinical judgements should be undertaken considering the research evidence base and the application of relevant research findings that complement the experiential (by doing) learning that clinical exposure has provided.

Following the guidance of the CoP student paramedics and paramedics undertaking higher education programmes will find that all curricula contain research

Paramedic Academic level 5 Dip HE, Foundation degree	Specialist paramedic Academic level 6 BSc Honours degree, graduate certificate or diploma	Advanced paramedic Academic level 7 Master's degree, post-graduate certificate or diploma	Consultant paramedic Academic level 8 Doctorate
May evaluate equipment, techniques and procedures May undertake straightforward or complex audit or assist with clinical trials or research projects	May also carry out research and development (R&D) as a major activity. May regularly undertake clinical trials or research projects	As specialist role but may in addition initiate and develop R&D programmes.	As advanced practice role but may in addition coordinate and implement R&D programmes and/or initiate and develop programmes with external impact

Figure 1.1 Paramedic career frameworks: research and development (adapted from College of Paramedics 2008: 20)

appreciation and the student's ability to critique research papers will be assessed. Furthermore, within essays and other assignments it will be necessary to demonstrate understanding of the research process and utilise informed discussion of published research papers. This emphasis on research for the educational preparation of the paramedic is so they can 'use research evidence to design, improve and implement effective paramedic practice' (CoP 2008: 53) and thus to, importantly, improve patient outcomes. Paramedics and paramedic students must develop an enduring curiosity for knowledge and a commitment to the appraisal and development of paramedic practice. This requires individual review of practice and, increasingly, consideration and critique of what is accepted practice. The Paramedic Career Framework (CoP 2008) notes that involvement with research and development is a core element of paramedics' professional development towards a future where consultant paramedics lead the profession's evolution (see Figure 1.1).

About this book

This book seeks to give the paramedic student, and the registered paramedic who is new to research, an introductory overview of key elements of research, providing sufficient information and guidance to further reading so that the paramedic is enabled to engage with research to inform and develop clinical practice. For paramedics undertaking programmes at Master's level that require a research to be undertaken, this book will give basic skills in developing and conducting a research study that will then be complemented with more specific methodological reading. It may be that the book will simply aid the inquiring paramedic, who is seeking to research an aspect of their own practice, a clear overview of how to go about it.

What is research?

When we use the term research we usually consider the systematic processes used to investigate something that we know little or even nothing about. Usually the knowledge generated will then contribute to an existing body of knowledge related to that particular topic. During the course of this book you will be introduced to different ways of collecting data (methods) and the philosophical underpinnings of these methods (methodology). We consider someone actively involved in carrying out research as being 'research active'; however, all paramedics must be 'research minded'. To be research minded is to be seeking consciously to ask questions of practice that can be answered by research. This can be through seeking out research conducted by others either by reviewing published papers or consulting systematic reviews of research studies often presented in guidelines such as those produced by the National Institute for Health and Clinical Excellence (NICE) or the Joint Royal Colleges Ambulance Liaison Committee (JRCALC).

What is a profession?

The paramedic profession became a registered occupation in 2000 when paramedics were required to register with the Council of Professions Supplementary to Medicine, an organisation that became the Health Professions Council (HPC) (Donaghy 2008). To move to full professional status certain criteria must be satisfied. Flexner's classic 1915 essay 'Is social work a profession' (Flexner 1915/2001) stated six criteria for a profession:

1 Professional activity is based on intellectual action along with personal responsibility.

2 The practice of a profession is based on knowledge, not routine activities.

3 There is practical application rather than just theorising.

4 There are techniques that can be taught.

5 A profession is organised internally.

6 A profession is motivated by altruism, with members working in some sense for the good of society.

If you were to check Flexner's criteria and then estimate how many of them are achieved by the paramedic profession currently, what would you answer? Within this chapter we will consider the second criterion: the practice of a profession is based on knowledge, not routine activities.

Development of the paramedic role

The use of litters or horse-drawn carts to carry the ill or the dead was developed during the Bonaparte Wars in 1793 to provide transport and treatment for the wounded. This mode of transport was also used in the United Kingdom in the nineteenth century by the police to transport patients in hand-litters and municipal asylums had horse-drawn fever ambulances. Motor vehicles classified as ambulances were used during the two World Wars (Claggs and Blaber 2008).

By the 1960s the ambulance driver's role was to transfer patients between home and hospital. Minimal training was received and requirements for the role were to be able to drive, to be strong and, predominantly, to be a man. Over time it was realised that basic emergency care could be provided by ambulance services and ambulance drivers received rudimentary first aid training, but it still remained a low status and semi-skilled job. The Millar Report (Ministry of Health 1966) recommended that ambulance training should be delivered in a more consistent manner and required that a minimal level of equipment be provided on ambulances. Despite this development, preparation for ambulance personnel remained short and relied on a training delivery rather than an educational approach (CoP 2008). This training focussed on rote delivery, where learning is by routine or repetition, often without full comprehension of the topic and with limited ability to transfer or to question learning. This degree of inflexibility resulted in limited ability to respond to new demands facing the service (Brady and Haddow (in press)). From the 1970s, changes in emergency care provision especially improvements in advanced life support, including defibrillation and resuscitation of severe trauma, gave ambulance personnel an increasingly enhanced role resulting in the registered title of paramedic in 2000. The learning approach remained, however, that of training rather than of education.

The Institute of Health and Care Delivery (IHCD) ambulance technician training developed from the Millar certified course to prepare ambulance technicians and paramedics was the method of paramedic preparation prior to the entry of paramedic education into higher education. These courses were short and involved much learning 'on the job' whilst employed as a technician or a paramedic trainee. The management of immediately life-threatening medical conditions and trauma management were the major educational content of these programmes (Brady and Haddow (in press)). It had become clear however that the 'blue light' high drama aspect of the paramedic work experience had led the content of ambulance training whereas the majority of calls are not in fact life threatening (CoP 2008). In *Taking Healthcare to the Patient: Transforming NHS Ambulance Services* (DH 2005), (known as the Bradley report), it was suggested that the paramedic should provide a wider range of emergency and unscheduled care and should offer interventions to assist patients to remain at home and so not require admission to hospital. Furthermore, paramedics should be prepared educationally for their role within a higher education setting using curricula guided by the CoP and developed and delivered in partnerships with paramedic NHS Trusts. This new curriculum would prepare the paramedic for developing roles and enhance adaptability. In *High Quality Care for All* (Darzi 2008) a vision of appropriate care being delivered where needed was offered:

> *Partnership working between the NHS, local authorities and social care partners will help to improve people's health and wellbeing, by organising services around patients, and not people around services.* (Darzi 2008: 43)

The paramedic profession is responding to the educational and the political challenges to provide care centred on patient needs rather than the needs of the organisation. The roles and responsibilities of ambulance and paramedic practitioners have therefore broadened in response to developments in medical care, societal change and political initiatives. The need for paramedics to be able to respond effectively to this reality required a new approach to their educational development in that learning must be a lifelong process and that on-going professional and personal continuous development was essential. The Quality Assurance Agency (QAA) benchmarks statements for paramedic practice note that:

> *The development of the reflective practitioner with a commitment to continuing professional development is fostered by developing a research ethic to contribute to the research portfolio in order to enhance the scientific base of the profession, improve patient care and optimise professional autonomy.* (QAA 2004: 7)

Professional autonomy carries a high expectation of professional accountability. This requires that the professional be held responsible for any acts or omissions that may cause the patient harm if that harm was due to the paramedic lacking knowledge or skills that it would be reasonable to expect them to have.

Knowledge to inform paramedic practice

Paramedic training and practice has been guided by the Joint Royal Colleges Ambulance Liaison Committee (JRCALC) since 1989. JRCALC UK Ambulance Service Clinical Practice guidelines are developed, or updated, on a five-year cycle based on systematic reviews of the evidence and consensus agreement to provide ambulance services with clear robust clinical guidance. These guidelines are drawn up by a committee that comprises paramedic and other professional bodies, in particular the medical Royal Colleges, with a three-yearly meeting hosted by the Royal College of Anaesthetists in London (JRCALC 2011). Increasingly paramedics are taking greater ownership of the knowledge base of their profession but this knowledge remains medically dependent currently. The challenge for the paramedic profession is to develop its own body of knowledge whilst drawing on other professional knowledge as appropriate.

Future knowledge

The paramedic practising in the twenty-first century has knowledge and skills that are quite unrecognisable from the transporting function of the early ambulance driver. The paramedic is required to exercise professional autonomy and deliver high level interventions in difficult circumstances. The UK-wide modernisation agenda (DH 2005) notes that a common educational framework should be delivered within higher education with its curriculum guided by the College of Paramedics/British Paramedic Association (2008) and the QAA (2004). The evolving role of the paramedic is reflected in the key changes to the CoP curriculum for paramedic registrant (CoP 2008) that notes that the paramedic should be skilled in:

- making appropriate referrals
- providing increased patient assessment

- undertaking enhanced history taking
- enhancing clinical decision making
- appreciating research and understanding research methodology.

These abilities cannot be learnt by rote but rather by having a critical understanding of the knowledge base of the paramedic profession, including learning from and in practice and using skills of reflection to aid this process of continuous learning (Rolfe et al. 2010).

Clinical decision making

Clinical decision making is a useful catch-all term to explain the practice of the health professional. When confronted with a patient the clinician has to:

- assess the situation
- develop a working *hypothesis* or idea of just what the issue/problem is
- collect more information to confirm or disprove the initial impression
- put in place interventions
- evaluate the effectiveness of the interventions
- reassess if required.

This problem solving approach is used by all health professionals (Higgs et al. 2008) including paramedics. The paramedic draws on past knowledge (theoretical and experiential) and the expert paramedic can often surprise the student paramedic by making what seems instant decisions even before all the assessment has been completed. To act as an autonomous professional clinical decision maker the paramedic must include best and current knowledge to inform their decisions: their practice must be evidence based.

Paramedic research

Paramedics have engaged in higher education since the 1990s as part of their post-qualifying continuous personal and professional development, undertaking Honours and Master's degrees and PhDs. However, the body of paramedic research conducted and led by paramedics in the UK remains limited. One notable example of a paramedic who has been involved in large numbers of funded research projects is one of the chapter authors of this book, Malcolm Woollard. See Box 1.1. You will note that this fairly recent study of paramedic practitioners has only one paramedic listed as an author. A key challenge to the evolving and inspirational paramedic research profile is to have more paramedics as leaders of such research projects.

Box 1.1 An example of a paramedic involved in research study into paramedic practice

Effectiveness of paramedic practitioners in attending 999 calls from elderly people in the community: cluster randomised controlled trial (Mason et al. 2007)

Authors:
Suzanne Mason, reader in emergency medicine
Emma Knowles, research fellow
Brigitte Colwell, research associate
Simon Dixon, senior lecturer
Jim Wardrope, consultant in emergency medicine
Robert Gorringe, lead emergency care practitioner
Helen Snooks, professor of health services research
Julie Perrin, nurse consultant in emergency medicine and Jon Nicholl, professor
One paramedic involved, Robert Gorringe, lead emergency care practitioner.

The profession's regulator, the Health Professions Council (HPC), (2007:9) requires that the registering paramedic should:

- recognise the value of research to the critical evaluation of practice

- be able to engage in evidence based practice, evaluate practice

- be aware of a range of research methodologies

- be able to demonstrate a logical and systematic approach to problem solving

- be able to evaluate research and other evidence to inform their own practice systematically and participate in audit procedures.

This level of research expertise remains that of a 'user' rather than that of a 'doer' of research; however, as we noted earlier, the Career Framework envisaged by the CoP sees paramedics engaging with and leading research. The readers of this book will probably be the generation of paramedic researchers that take control over their own profession, and the generation of that profession specific knowledge. Jones and Jones (2009) suggest that with increasing numbers of paramedics undertaking research proposals or small-scale research projects for their degrees this will lead to more paramedics publishing their work and so enhance the professional standing of the profession. This is to be commended.

Jones and Jones (2009) further highlight the conundrum facing those who seek to develop research undertaken by paramedics to inform paramedic practice in that, due to paramedic science being a relatively new discipline in higher education, those who often teach research to paramedics are not paramedics. Jones and Jones (2009: 467) suggest that: 'This perhaps limits their ability to provide adequate example or application of major research concepts to a practice situation which could be understood by the pre-hospital specialist'.

This concern can be countered by noting that higher education lecturers often lecture to many professional health groups. Good teaching practice requires that profession-specific research examples are utilised and that the students are guided to discover the relevance to their practice. Jones and Jones's comments are, however, pertinent and it is to be hoped that as paramedic research and education develops there will be an increasing number of paramedics who will be teaching research in higher education settings and who will also become leaders of research studies.

The research process: an overview

The research process is a framework to help the researcher plan research in a logical manner. Whereas it is often seen as a linear process, it certainly is not, often requiring the researcher to revisit certain aspects of the process. Below is an overview of the research process.

- *The aim or problem* – all researchers need to start off with an aim or problem which they wish to investigate and find an answer to. A paramedic for instance may notice a practice that seems illogical and wonder if it could be done better.

- *Ethical approval* – all researchers must consider the ethical issues that the study causes; in many cases ethical approval will need to be sought and gained from local ethics committees before the study can be carried out.

- *The literature review* – this is an important part of the research process. The researcher needs to review the literature to ascertain what research has already been carried out. It may be that the researcher could replicate a study, building on existing research findings. The literature may point the researcher in another direction or it may identify 'gaps' in the literature – areas where research has not yet been carried out. In some cases it may highlight that there is no need to carry out the proposed research. From critically reviewing the literature the researcher should be able to define the studies aims or questions to be addressed.

- *Research aim or questions* – the researcher should clearly outline the aim and objectives or research questions. The question will guide the appropriate methodology for the study.

- *The methodology and research design* – the researcher will describe the approach taken to undertake the study and whether a *qualitative* or *quantitative* approach will be used or if using both describe a mixed methodology. The researcher should choose the most appropriate research approach to answer the study aim(s), question(s) or hypothesis.

- *The sample* should be determined – outlining who or what the sample is, the size of the sample (which will also be determined by the approach taken), how the sample will be approached, and how the researcher will gain access to the sample.

- *Data collection tool(s)* – the methodological approach taken will determine whether a questionnaire, interview, observations, experiment or other approach will be used to collect the data.

- *Pilot study* – the pilot study is where the data collection tool and method of collection is carried out on a small sample who will not be involved in the main study. Researchers often make some changes to their data collection tool following the pilot study.

- *Data collection* – the method used will determine how the data will be collected. If the researcher is collecting qualitative data the researcher may interview research participants. If the researcher is collecting quantitative data they may use a questionnaire.

- *Data analysis* (or making sense of the data collected) – this stage of the research process should not be underestimated in the timescale that it will take to analysis the data and produce findings. If interviews have been used to collect qualitative data the interviews will have to be transcribed prior to analysis. Quantitative data will often be entered onto a spreadsheet. Quantitative researchers often use a computer program called SPSS (Statistical Package for the Social Sciences) to facilitate statistical analysis.

- *Discussion and conclusions*– the researcher will present the findings in a format identifying common themes (qualitative) or making statistical conclusions (quantitative) and relating findings to published literature. The researcher will draw conclusions from their study's findings and will make recommendations for practice, education and further research.

- *Dissemination* – this is a vital part of the research process. It is important that the researcher communicates their findings of the study through publications and/or presentations, locally and internationally.

Structure of this book

In Chapter 2 the nature of different forms of knowing involved in paramedic practice and the philosophical difference between qualitative and quantitative research approaches are discussed. The evidence based nature of paramedic practice is explored in Chapter 3. In Chapter 4 the key ethical considerations when undertaking research are considered. The conduct of a literature review is discussed in Chapter 5. In Chapters 6 and 7 an introduction to qualitative research is presented and Chapters 8 and 9 provide an introduction to quantitative research. In Chapter 10 advice on how to research clinical practice and practical recommendations on how to write for publication are offered. Chapter 11 completes the book and here future directions for paramedic research are considered.

Overall, this book provides an introduction to research and to the research process and we hope that reading this book will act as a springboard for the reader's informed use of research and to the conduct of research projects that shape paramedic practice.

References

Brady, M. and Haddow, P. (in press) Evolving education in paramedic practice. *Ambulance UK.*

Claggs, B. and Blaber, A. (2008) Consideration of history. In: Blaber, A. (ed.) *Foundations for Paramedic Practice. A Theoretical Approach.* Maidenhead: McGraw Hill/Open University Press, pp. 1–11.

College of Paramedics (2008) *Paramedic Curriculum Guidance and Competence Framework* (2nd edn). Derby: College of Paramedics.

Darzi, A. (2008) *High Quality Care for All. NHS Next Stage Review.* London: The Stationery Office.

Department of Health (2005) *Taking Healthcare to the Patient: Transforming NHS Ambulance Services.* London: DH.

Donaghy, J. (2008) Higher education for paramedics – why? *Journal of Paramedic Practice* 1(1): 31–35.

Flexner, A. ([1915] 2001) Is social work a profession? *Research on Social Work Practice* 11(2): 152–165.

Health Professions Council (2007) *Standards of Proficiency – Paramedics.* London: HPC.

Higgs, J., Jones, M.A. Loftus, S. and Christensen, N. (eds) (2008) *Clinical Reasoning in the Health Professions* (3rd edn). London: Butterworth Heinemann Elsevier.

Joint Royal Colleges Ambulance Liaison Committee (JRCALC). *Guidelines.* Available at: http://jrcalc.org.uk/guidelines.html [accessed 20 March 2011].

Jones, C. and Jones, P. (2009) Paramedic research method: importance and implications. *Journal of Paramedic Practice* 1(11): 465–469.

Mason, S., Knowles, E., Colwell, B. et al. (2007) Effectiveness of paramedic practitioners in attending 999 calls to elderly people in the community: cluster randomised controlled trial. *British Medical Journal* 19 doi: 10.1136/bmj.39343.649097.55. Available at: http://www.bmj.com/content/335/7626/919.abstract [accessed 17 April 2011].

Ministry of Health Scottish Home and Health Department (1966) *Report by the Working Party on Ambulance Training and Equipment.* London: Ministry of Health.

Rolfe, G., Freshwater, D. and Jasper, M. (2010) *Critical Reflection for Nursing and the Helping Professions. A User's Guide* (2nd edn). Basingstoke: Palgrave.

Quality Assurance Agency (QAA) (2004) *Benchmarking Statement for Paramedic Science.* Gloucester: QAA.

2 Knowledge to underpin paramedic practice

Gary Rolfe

Learning outcomes for the chapter
By the end of this chapter the reader should be able to:

1   Identify and appreciate the importance of a variety of different types of knowledge for practice

2   Understand the basic differences between qualitative and quantitative and mixed-methods approaches to research

3   Understand the importance and relevance of different ontological and epistemo-logical theories in determining which research approach to employ

4   Understand the importance of critique and recognise and differentiate between different levels and purposes

Keywords
epistemological
knowledge
qualitative
quantitative

The nature of knowledge

Imagine the following scenario: an ambulance crew of two paramedics were called to attend a 30-year-old woman named Alice, known to them from previous visits. While on the way to the job, the crew was informed by ambulance control that Alice was discovered by her partner, having made cuts to both wrists, and it was he who had made the call to the emergency services. They briefly discussed what they were likely to find on arrival and decided which aspects of the job each of them would attend to. When they arrived, the crew was greeted by Alice's partner, who explained that he came home early from work to find her semi-conscious and bleeding profusely from both wrists. They knew immediately that, unlike on their previous calls to this patient, she had severed both radial arteries and appeared to be in shock. While one crew member spoke with Alice's partner, the other quickly applied pressure to both wrists. They then transferred her to the ambulance, where they set up an intravenous line. On the journey to the hospital they spoke with Alice and her partner about the incident, and by the time they had reached the accident and emergency (A&E) department they had discovered that, in addition to cutting her wrists, Alice had also taken an overdose of paracetamol. This information was conveyed to the senior registrar on arrival at the A&E department, and the crew took a brief break to talk about the case before their next call.

Although this was a routine call for this experienced ambulance crew, the range of different types of knowledge that they required in order to ensure a safe and effective outcome was anything but simple. They already knew a great deal about the situation they were being called to before they had even arrived. They knew Alice personally from a number of previous calls from her for attempted suicide and self-harm; they knew that she had made cuts to her wrists and they knew that, unlike on previous occasions, it was not Alice herself who had informed the emergency services. They had also anticipated certain other aspects of the situation such as the likely mental state of Alice's partner and had agreed upon a strategy for dealing with it.

Immediately upon arrival at Alice's flat they could see that the wounds were deep, that Alice had already lost a great deal of blood, and that she was semi-conscious, apparently from shock. They knew the procedures to be followed in such a case and they knew how to implement them. They also correctly anticipated that her partner was extremely distressed and they knew that he would need to be calmed down before the trip to the hospital. They also knew that the more information they could hand over on arrival at the A&E department, the better would be the prognosis for the patient, and so they continued to talk with Alice and her partner during the journey to hospital. They then took a little time to review the case and to think about what had gone well and not so well, and to relax before their next job. They knew themselves and each other well enough to be able to quickly put themselves back in the right frame of mind to carry on with their work.

If we think more closely about all the different types of knowledge that the ambulance crew possessed and used before, during and after this call, we will see that there was a great deal more involved in achieving a successful outcome than simply recognising that the patient had cut her wrists and knowing the correct procedure to implement. In fact, we can break down the wide variety of different kinds of knowledge that the crew brought to the job into four types.

Knowing-that

Firstly, they brought with them a huge fund of medical, anatomical, sociological and psychological knowledge. This included knowledge about the anatomy and physiology of the arm and its veins, arteries, nerves and ligaments, about the effects of blood loss on the body and brain, about patterns of behaviour in suicide and self-harm attempts, and about the psychological effects on the patient and on loved ones of attempted suicide. For example, they knew *that* a severed artery would result in significant blood loss and eventual death, they knew *that* the patient would lose consciousness due to a lack of oxygen to the brain, they knew *that* a change in Alice's usual pattern of self-harm attempts might have some significance (although they did not know at this stage quite what it might signify), and they knew *that* the impact of discovering Alice would probably have a psychological and even physical effect on her partner (although they might not know precisely what form the effect would take). Much of this knowledge is freely available in textbooks and research papers, and would have been acquired by the ambulance crew mostly through a combination of reading and attending lectures. This type of knowledge, which we will refer to here as *knowing-that*, is also sometimes called theoretical knowledge or *propositional knowledge*, since it is largely *generalisable* and can be expressed in words in the form of propositions or statements about the world.

Knowing-how

Secondly, the crew brought with them a fund of practical know-how. This included knowing *how* to apply pressure to a bleeding wound, knowing *how* to set up a drip, knowing *how* to calm down a distressed relative and knowing *how* to gain the trust of Alice and her partner in order to encourage them to talk about the incident. Some of this knowledge, including most of the first aid and medical procedures, would have been learnt in the classroom or in a simulated practice setting, but some, such as knowing how to calm people down and knowing how to gain their trust, would have been accumulated over time from previous practice situations.

Knowing-why

In straightforward and routine cases, it is often sufficient to know the general theory of what to do and the standard procedures for how to do it. However, most practitioners will sooner or later come across a case that is not routine and for which the general procedure does not work. For example, whereas the procedure for staunching heavy blood flow is compression to the site of the wound, there will be some cases where, for a variety of reasons, compression will be neither desirable nor practical. In some of these cases there might well be alternative procedures, but there will always be unique one-off cases where there is no written protocol and no relevant prior experience to draw upon. In such cases, the practitioner must think on-the-spot and come up with a unique solution to meet the needs of the unique situation, and this demands not only knowing *that* a certain procedure is usually followed and knowing *how* to implement the procedure, but also knowing *why* it is followed. It is only by understanding *why*, for example, a tourniquet is not usually applied to prevent bleeding that the practitioner might safely and effectively apply one in exceptional circumstances. A practitioner who has merely been trained in the 'correct' procedure without any understanding of *why* it is correct will not have the resources to try something different when the correct procedure cannot be employed.

Knowing-who

We can see from the above example that the paramedics knew not only what to do, why it was the right thing to do, and how to do it, but they also had some limited knowledge of *who* they were doing it to. In this case they had the rare

Table 2.1 Summary of ways of knowing

Knowing-that	Theoretical knowledge found in books and research journals that can be widely applied to different situations
Knowing-how	Practical knowledge gained from training sessions and also from past experience
Knowing-why	A deeper understanding of a situation that allows practitioners to work outside of standard procedures
Knowing-who	Personal knowledge of other people and ourselves that enables practitioners to apply general knowing-that and knowing-how to specific and unique cases

advantage of having had previous contact with the patient, although most crews on most jobs will arrive with some rudimentary social and demographic knowledge of the person they are dealing with, if only their gender and approximate age. Furthermore, unless the patient is unconscious, there is generally an opportunity to acquire more knowledge about the patient by talking to them during treatment and en route to hospital. It is also important that practitioners know themselves and each other and how they are likely to respond to and cope with the stressful and often distressing situations that they will be encountering on a regular basis.

Although this *knowing-who* might appear to be 'soft' knowledge compared to the more technical *knowing-that*, *knowing-how* and *knowing-why*, it is worth recalling that, in the above example, the *knowing-who* was of crucial importance. It was through getting to know Alice as a person that the crew was able to recognise that this particular suicide attempt was different from previous ones made by the same patient, which in turn led the crew to the discovery that she had also taken a paracetamol overdose. Arguably, then, a purely technical intervention might have saved the life of the patient in the short term, only for her to die of liver failure two or three days later. See Table 2.1.

Knowledge and practice

Although these four types of knowledge have been presented and discussed separately, they are usually applied in parallel or alternated in quick succession in real-life clinical situations. For example, the potentially life-saving disclosure by Alice that she had taken an overdose came about as the result of the application of all four types of knowledge. The paramedic used his *knowing-who* about Alice, gained from his previous acquaintance with her, to recognise that this suicide attempt did not follow the usual pattern of her calling the emergency services following superficial cuts to her wrist. This led him to the hypothesis that she might this time be more serious in her intent. He used his *knowing-that* to draw on theories of suicide taught to him during his pre- or post-registration educational programmes which suggest that more than one method is often used in serious attempts, and his theoretical knowledge from reading a textbook that the effects of paracetamol overdose are often not noticeable for up to 24 hours. He used his *knowing-how* to gain the trust of Alice through counselling techniques that he had learned at a workshop and which he had refined and modified through previous experience. As this was not a standard counselling setting, he used his theoretical *knowing-why* to modify his counselling interventions to suit the situation, which enabled Alice to feel safe enough to disclose to him that she had taken an overdose. Perhaps most importantly, he used his insights about his own psychology, his *knowing-who* he was as a person, to ensure that his own negative feelings about what he sometimes referred to as 'time wasters' did not cause him to dismiss this suicide attempt as superficial. What therefore appeared to the casual observer to be a simple and straightforward chat in the back of an ambulance actually entailed the application of a great deal of specialised and detailed knowledge about the theory and practice of paramedic science.

How practice knowledge is generated

Having explored the kinds of knowledge required for safe and effective practice, we will now turn our attention to how this knowledge is generated. As we shall see, some practice knowledge seems to require little or no effort on our part, some comes about through thinking and experimenting during practice itself, and some is generated systematically through research projects. See Table 2.2.

Intuitive knowing

Some *knowing-how* and *knowing-who* is acquired naturally and without conscious thought by practitioners themselves simply through repeating an experience many times. For example, the knowledge of how to talk to distressed patients is often accumulated and refined over time without any formal training. Similarly, many experienced practitioners report that they can recognise certain medical problems straight away without any conscious thought or consideration. Dreyfus and Dreyfus (1986) regarded this ability to *just know* certain things without having to think about them as the defining characteristic of *expert practice*, and claimed that the expert practitioner is unconsciously matching certain features of the present situation with similar features of situations that had been encountered and successfully resolved in the past. Dreyfus and Dreyfus claimed that this 'pattern matching'

Table 2.2 Sources of knowledge for practice

Intuitive knowing	Knowing the right thing to do without fully realising how or why you know it. Intuitive knowing can be acquired unconsciously or through reflecting-on-action
Knowing-in-practice	Gaining an understanding of practice whilst it is happening. Knowing-in-practice can be acquired through reflection-in-action or more formally through small-scale action research
Research-based knowledge	Knowledge from formal research projects that involve systematic and rigorous inquiry

was an intuitive process that did not follow any rules and could not be expressed in words. As they pointed out:

> In reality, a patient is viewed by the experienced doctor as a unique case and treated on the basis of intuitively perceived similarity with situations previously encountered. That kind of wisdom, unfortunately, cannot be shared and thereby made the basis of a doctor's rational decision. (Dreyfus and Dreyfus 1986: 200)

Thus, when asked why she responded in the way she did to a distressed patient, the expert paramedic would often not be able to say, nor would she be able to pass on this *tacit knowledge* to colleagues and students.

Although Dreyfus and Dreyfus described this form of expert knowing as 'understanding without a rationale', Schön (1983) believed that at least some aspects of it could be articulated and understood through a process of *reflection on action* that involved the practitioner consciously thinking back about how her clinical decisions were made. In this way, not only could the rationale for the decisions be explored and examined, but theories could be constructed in order to make sense of what appeared at the time as intuitive or spontaneous action. For example, if the practitioner was asked to reflect in a systematic way on what she was thinking and feeling whilst counselling a distressed patient, Schön believed that in some situations the practitioner would be able to explain and pass on her rationale in the form of knowledge and theory. In other words, he suggested that reflection on action enables practitioners to generate and describe *knowing-that* and *knowing-why* to explain their tacit *knowing-how* and *knowing-who*.

Knowing-in-practice

More importantly, however, Schön believed that it is possible to generate practice knowledge by reflecting *during* rather than after practice. Even while they are practising, practitioners are able to ask themselves questions such as:

- What features do I notice when I recognise this thing?

- What are the criteria by which I make this judgement?

- What procedures am I enacting when I perform this skill?

- How am I framing the problem that I am trying to solve?

(Schön 1983: 50)

Schön referred to this ability to 'turn thought back on action' as *reflection in action* and described it as a form of on-the-spot experimenting, such that 'when someone reflects-in-action he becomes a researcher in the practice context' (Schön 1983). Schön was therefore suggesting that, in certain situations, practice can be a form of research. Other writers have referred to this as action research or *practitioner research*, that is, research conducted by practitioners themselves as part of their practice (Fox et al. 2007).

Practitioner research of the kind described by Schön and others is an important and valuable way of generating knowledge from practice. However, the knowledge it produces is somewhat restricted; it is useful for understanding and resolving the problem that the practitioner is facing at the time, but it has limited usefulness for practice as a whole. For example, the paramedic in our earlier example was able to build up a store of *knowing-who* Alice was as a person that added to his *knowing-why* her suicide attempt might this time be more serious, which in turn led eventually to his *knowing-that* she had also taken an overdose of paracetamol. Whilst this knowledge might have been life-saving in this particular situation, it would be of little use either to that particular practitioner or to others in future situations with different patients.

Research based knowledge

It is now widely accepted that best practice needs to be based on evidence from formal research projects (Aveyard and Sharp 2009). In its simplest form, practice research can be defined as 'the systematic and rigorous process of inquiry which aims to … contribute to a scientific body of knowledge' (Bowling 2009: 16). Most definitions of research emphasise that the findings should be generalisable to other settings and populations, and whilst the intuitive knowing as described by Dreyfus and Dreyfus and the knowing-in-practice as described by Schön are both important to paramedic practice, neither can be described as research based according to this definition. Intuitive knowledge is not derived from a 'systematic and rigorous process of inquiry', and whilst the methods used to generate knowing-in-practice might, in some cases, be described as systematic, we have seen that the outcome does not 'contribute to a scientific body of knowledge' that can be employed by other practitioners and generalised to other situations. The focus of the remainder of this chapter is therefore on more formal and structured research projects.

Qualitative and quantitative paradigms

We have seen that paramedic practice requires a wide variety of different types of knowing, ranging from general scientific theories to very personal knowledge about ourselves and our individual patients. Paramedic practice research therefore employs a wide range of methods and methodologies from a variety of different academic and practice disciplines.

The different methods and methodologies employed in practice research are often categorised as either qualitative or quantitative depending on whether the data they generate takes the form of words or numbers. However, the common feature of all of these research methods and methodologies is, as the above definition suggests, an emphasis on a systematic and rigorous process. Most researchers believe that it is only through rigorously adhering to particular methods that the validity and *reliability* of the findings can be ensured.

The qualitative methods employed in paramedic research mostly derive from anthropology and other social sciences, and include structured and unstructured interviews and participant and non-participant observations. Other qualitative methods such as autobiographical and reflective writing originate in the disciplines of philosophy and literature, whilst some of the more participative methods such as cooperative inquiry and action research are taken from practice disciplines such as education and nursing. The quantitative methods of data collection employed in

Table 2.3 Types of research

Approach	Some typical methods and methodologies
Qualitative	Structured interviews
	Unstructured interviews
	Participant observation
	Non-participant observation
	Autobiographical writing
	Reflective writing
	Action research
Quantitative	Tick-box questionnaires
	Attitude and opinion scales
	Randomised controlled trials

paramedic research are drawn mainly from the disciplines of sociology and psychology, and include tick-box *survey* questionnaires, some forms of non-participant observation and numerical attitude and opinion scales. All of these methods will be discussed in more detail later in the book. More recently, and partly in response to the evidence based practice movement (see Chapter 3), *experimental research* has gained in prominence. As we shall see in later chapters, experimental methods such as the randomised controlled trial have been adapted from their origins in agricultural and medical research to provide a methodology for demonstrating causal relationships and for making direct statistical comparisons between different treatments. See Table 2.3.

How do you choose which method to use?

To some extent the choice of a qualitative or quantitative method would depend on the research question being asked. If we want to know the *quantity* of patients seen by the ambulance service last year we will almost certainly use a quantitative method, whereas if we want to know what the patients thought about the *quality* of the service we are more likely to employ a qualitative method.

In some cases, however, the choice between a qualitative and a quantitative approach is not quite so straightforward. For example, we could discover patients' opinions of the ambulance service either by asking them to describe it to us in their own words or by asking them to rate it on a scale from one to ten. Each approach will provide us with data about the quality of the service, but the former uses a qualitative method and the latter uses a quantitative method. In this case, our choice of method will be based not only on the research question but also on the type of knowledge that we wish to generate. For example, if we are interested in *knowing-that* the service is meeting the expectations of the patients, we might ask them to rate it numerically from one to ten. We can then show on a graph which aspects of the service are performing well and which sections of the population are happy with it. If, on the other hand, we are interested in *knowing-why* certain aspects of the service are not meeting the expectations of the population, we might ask patients to describe the service in their own words. Sometimes we might want both types of information: often we would begin by wishing to know *that* something was or was not the case and then move on to discover *why* it might be so. This might require a combination of quantitative and qualitative approaches known as *mixed-methods* or multi-method research.

Philosophical underpinnings

Whilst some researchers see a multi-methods strategy as a practical commonsense way of producing broad and varied knowledge for practice (Cresswell and Plano-Clark 2010), others believe that qualitative and quantitative approaches are fundamentally different and should not be used together in the same study. For these researchers, the terms 'qualitative' and 'quantitative' do not merely describe data collection methods, but are shorthand terms for two different philosophies about the nature of knowledge (*epistemology*) and even the nature of reality (*ontology*).

Realism – what you see is what you get

The philosophy on which quantitative research is based is usually known as *realism*. In simple terms, realists believe that 'what you see is what you get', that the external world is directly present to us and that, under normal circumstances, we all have more or less undistorted access to reality. When I look at a tree, I see more or less what you see when you look at the same tree, and we are in more or less total agreement about what it is we are both looking at. That is not to say that we are not sometimes fooled by illusions, delusions and hallucinations, but rather that we accept that, behind the illusion, there is a real tree that we are all able to perceive in much the same way.

For realists, the purpose of research is to provide us with clear and undistorted access to the real world so that we can measure, categorise and record it. Our tools for gaining access to the reality or the truth of the world are our five senses, and the purpose of empirical scientific research is to provide us with a method for observing the world in as clear and undistorted a way as possible. The scientific method therefore attempts to minimise internal distortion by insisting on an objective, controlled and detached stance on the part of the researcher, and minimises external distortion by careful selection of the research subjects, by ensuring that the data collection tools measure consistently and accurately what they were designed to measure, and by minimising the influence and impact of the research on the research setting and subjects. For this reason, the accuracy and precision of numerical data is usually preferred to words, which are more open to subjective interpretation by the researcher.

Constructionism – what you see is what you have been taught to see

Whilst the realist claim that there is a 'real world' directly available to our senses might appear little more than common sense, *constructionism* disputes this straightforward view of the world and our knowledge of it. Constructionists believe that we can have no immediate and direct access to the real world, but that all of our perceptions are socially constructed. A newborn baby would therefore not see a tree at all, but would perceive a shifting pattern of green and brown that would be indistinguishable from the background and from the objects around it. A tree only becomes a distinct object in its own right when the child is taught what a tree is. Similarly, whereas a botanist might see a mature horse chestnut, a child would only see a generic tree, or possibly a source of conkers. We always perceive the world through one or more social or theoretical lens, so that, as the poet and artist William Blake ([1793] 2010) put it, 'A fool sees not the same tree that a wise man sees'.

Unlike the realists, who regard the purpose of research as providing undistorted access to reality, the constructionists consider this to be a more or less impossible task. There is, of course, a real physical world 'out there', but all our knowledge of it is subjective, which is to say, the very act of perceiving the world introduces the social, cultural and personal bias of the person who is making the observation. The quantitative research *paradigm*, where data are represented as numbers, might give the illusion of producing objective scientific knowledge, but presenting the attitudes or opinions of people in numerical form is no less of a distorted and subjective interpretation of what they 'really' think than it would be to ask them to describe their opinions qualitatively in their own words. Thus, whereas the task of the realist researcher is to ensure objectivity by keeping separate the views, opinions and interventions of researcher from what is being researched, the constructionist researcher recognises that the researcher and the researched are intimately connected even before the research study has commenced. Objectivity is impossible, and the very best that the constructionist can do is to recognise, monitor and document their own involvement and influence on the production of the data.

As a rough guide, most quantitative researchers subscribe (sometimes without realising it) to realism, although a growing number are describing themselves as critical realists, a philosophical position midway between realism and constructionism. On the other hand, most qualitative researchers tend to hold views more in line with constructionism, although the degree to which they accept or reject objectivity varies from one methodology to another. For example, some phenomenologists try to 'bracket' their own subjective preconceptions in order to be as objective as possible, whereas other schools of phenomenology encourage and celebrate the subjectivity of the researcher, arguing that it is an essential part of the research process. Other qualitative researchers, usually known as action researchers, abandon completely the distinction between research and practice and aim to bring about changes to practice as part of the process of doing research (Coghlan and Brannick 2010). This approach is in complete opposition to the traditional scientific research approach, where the researcher goes to great pains to avoid exerting any influence whatsoever on what or who is being observed or measured.

Inductivism – building a theory

The other main point of philosophical difference between qualitative and quantitative researchers concerns how they develop knowledge into a theory. Almost all qualitative researchers and some quantitative researchers adopt the method of inductivism, whereby they build theories from the ground up by accumulating a number of individual facts until enough is known about the subject to confidently base practice on it. For example, if a researcher wished to test the safety of a particular paramedic intervention, she might observe a number of instances of the intervention until she considered that she had accumulated enough cases to demonstrate that it was safe. In qualitative research, the exact number of observations required is not usually fixed in advanced, and observations would continue until *data saturation* has been reached, that is, until no new information is emerging. In quantitative research, the 'sample size' is often set in advance, either pragmatically or through a statistical calculation.

Hypothetico-deductivism – demolishing a theory

However, there is a fundamental flaw in inductive reasoning, since however many cases of safe interventions we might accumulate, it would take only a single observation of an unsafe intervention to destroy our theory. Taken to its logical conclusion, this 'problem of induction' (see, for example, Cardinal et al. 2004: 66) means that we can never be sure of anything, which prompted the philosopher Karl Popper (2002) to suggest an alternative to inductivism known as *hypothetico-deductivism*. Whereas inductive research gradually builds a theory that fits with the data that is being accumulated, hypothetico-deductive research proposes a tentative theory (sometimes called a hypothesis) at the outset of the study and then sets out to test whether it is likely to be true. We have seen that a theory can never conclusively be proved to be true, regardless of how much positive data we accumulate, but that a single piece of negative data can disprove it. We can never prove that a particular paramedic intervention is safe, regardless of how many safe interventions we witness, but we can *disprove* the theory that it is safe by finding a single instance where it was found to be unsafe.

The aim of hypothetico-deductivism is therefore to attempt to *disprove* theories by deliberately setting out to find negative instances. In the language of research, this entails deriving a *null hypothesis* from the theory, that is, to state the very opposite of what we hope our research will achieve. In the above example, the null hypothesis would be that the intervention is unsafe, and the research project would entail trying to disprove this null hypothesis by setting up as many potentially unsafe situations as possible. If, after we have subjected our intervention to the most extreme tests possible, we have not witnessed any examples of unsafe practice, we have good reason to reject our null hypothesis and consider the intervention to be safe. We still cannot be certain that it is safe, but we now have a great deal more confidence in it after our extreme testing than we would have done had it been subjected to an inductive research study that merely collected in a naturalistic way whatever data happened to come along. This approach of setting up controlled artificial situations for research rather than simply observing the world in its natural state is called experimentation, which will be discussed in much greater detail in later chapters.

Core elements of research studies

Literature reviews

Regardless of whether the study employs qualitative or quantitative methods of data collection, whether it is inductive or deductive, and whether it uses an experimental or a naturalistic design, the research process follows a relatively standard format. Most studies begin with a broad research aim or question that is refined and focussed by reviewing the existing relevant literature. The literature review fulfils the dual purpose firstly of identifying what has already been explored and achieved in the particular field and secondly of identifying where gaps in knowledge might exist that would warrant further study. It could be that, as a result of the literature review, we discover that our particular study has already been carried out, in which case the research question will need to be modified or even abandoned. On the other hand, the review might reveal that little or nothing has been achieved in relation to the research question, which could open up the opportunity for an entire programme of research. It is important that the review of the literature takes a critical perspective, since even if research has already been conducted in similar areas to our own, it is possible that its scope is limited or even that it is methodologically flawed.

Reasons for conducting a literature review

- to identify what has already been written on the topic
- to see whether similar studies have already been conducted
- to critically evaluate the usefulness, relevance and scientific merit of previous studies
- to identify gaps in the literature which a new study might fill
- to identify research tools and methods which have proved effective in the past.

Study design

Following the literature review, we are now in a position to focus our research aim or question and to develop from it a number of specific objectives or null hypotheses. We might already have decided on our research methodology and data collection methods, but it is more usual to select the most appropriate methodology to suit our question and to choose a method compatible with our methodology. For this reason, most research studies include a short section on the research methodology, including a rationale for why it was chosen, a brief outline of the philosophical position and a discussion about the ethical issues that it raises and how they are to be addressed. This is usually followed by a detailed description of the methods of sample selection, data collection and data analysis. It is very important that research studies go into a great deal of detail about how the study was conducted, since a rigorous adherence to the correct methodological procedures is important in the generation of valid and reliable research findings.

Findings

Having reviewed the relevant literature and discussed how we designed the study and collected the data, the next stage is to report on the findings. If we are conducting a quantitative study, the findings section will include statistical tables and usually a visual representation of the numerical data in the form of charts or graphs. If our study is qualitative, the findings section will include verbatim extracts from our transcripts. As well as presenting our findings, this section will usually explain and expand on our data and tentatively begin to discuss its relevance.

Discussion

This discussion is continued and elaborated upon in the next stage of the research process, where our findings are related back to our research question and to the wider literature. Questions to be addressed in this discussion section include:

- Did we find what we expected to find?

- Do our findings agree with or contradict the existing literature?

- Have we answered our research questions?

The discussion section might also include a critical reflection on our study to identify any limitations or omissions by posing questions such as:

- Did the design and conduct of our study limit its reliability and validity in any way?

- Was the chosen design the best or most appropriate to answer the research question?

- Was the study conducted in a way that produced valid and reliable findings?

Finally, it is usual to make recommendations both for practice and for further research.

Critiquing research

Knowledge comes in many forms and from many sources, and we have seen that scientific research is a particularly important source of knowledge for practice. However, the development of a discipline such as paramedic science requires more than simply the accumulation of more and more published research studies; all aspects of knowledge generation must be subject to critical analysis and judgement, an activity usually referred to as critique. Academic critique takes place on a number of levels (Rolfe 2008) as compiled in Table 2.4.

Conclusion

Even if paramedic practitioners are not directly involved in research projects, it is important for them to be able to read, understand and make critical judgements about the way that studies are conducted and the conclusions drawn from them. Evidence based practice demands that practitioners should review the scientific merit of research findings before applying them to practice, and this entails being able to understand the scientific and philosophical basis of different research

Table 2.4 Academic critiques

Critique of individual research studies	Focussed on whether a suitable and accepted methodology and method has been used, and the extent to which the rules of that particular methodology have been rigorously followed. The aim of this form of critique is to establish the validity and reliability of the study
Critique of methods and methodologies	Focussed on the suitability of the method and/or methodology for answering the research question
Critique of research paradigm	Focussed on whether the qualitative or quantitative paradigm is best suited for doing research within a particular discipline or field of practice

methods and methodologies at a fairly sophisticated level. The following chapter will continue with the theme of evidence based practice and later chapters will consider qualitative and quantitative research methodologies in greater detail.

References

Aveyard, H. and Sharp, P. (2009) *A Beginner's Guide to Evidence Based Practice in Health and Social Care*. Maidenhead: Open University Press.

Blake, W. ([1793] 2010) *The Marriage of Heaven and Hell*. Oxford: Oxford University Press.

Bowling, A. (2009) *Research Methods in Health: Investigating Health and Health Services* (3rd edn). Maidenhead: Open University Press.

Cardinal, D., Hayward, J. and Jones, G. (2004) *Epistemology: The Theory of Knowledge*. London: John Murray.

Coghlan, D. and Brannick, T. (2010) *Doing Action Research in Your Own Organization*. London: Sage.

Cresswell, J.W. and Plano-Clark, V.L. (2010) *Designing and Conducting Mixed Methods Research* (2nd edn). Los Angeles: Sage.

Dreyfus, H.L. and Dreyfus, S.E. (1986) *Mind Over Machine*. New York: Macmillan.

Fox, M., Martin, P. and Green, G. (2007) *Doing Practitioner Research*. London: Sage.

Popper, K. (2002) *Conjectures and Refutations*. London: Routledge.

Rolfe, G. (2008) Nursing and the art of radical critique. *Nurse Education Today* 28: 1–7.

Schön, D. (1983) *The Reflective Practitioner*. London: Temple Smith.

3 Evidence based practice in paramedic practice

Megan Rosser

Learning outcomes for the chapter

By the end of this chapter the reader should be able to:

1 Define evidence based practice and what constitutes evidence

2 Discuss the perceived benefits and challenges of evidence based practice

3 Describe the stages involved in implementing evidence based practice

4 Discuss the applicability of evidence based practice to paramedic practice and the challenges that practitioners might face

Keywords

clinical governance
clinical guidelines
evidence based practice

Introduction

As discussed in Chapter 2, the paramedic practitioner uses a variety of sources of knowledge but increasingly the paramedic is required to deliver care that has a sound evidence base. The phrase evidence based practice (EBP) or variations on that phrase have become increasingly commonplace in healthcare since the early 1990s. A number of government documents and policy drivers in the 1990s (DH 1997, 1998) raised the profile of evidence based practice in order to deliver high quality equitable and prompt care to patients that was also effective and efficient. The push behind this approach was to encourage practitioners to question their practice rather than continue to provide care that may have been provided for years without scrutiny or analysis. All practitioners, including paramedics, were encouraged to incorporate relevant, quality research findings into their practice rather than rely on anecdotal evidence.

The purpose of this chapter is to introduce you to the principles of evidence based practice and to enable you to apply these principles to paramedic practice.

Definitions of evidence based practice

Initially the concepts of evidence based practice were most closely applied to medicine, hence one of the earliest and most familiar definitions relates to medicine. Sackett et al. defined evidence based medicine as:

> *The conscientious, explicit and judicious use of current best evidence in making decisions about the care of the individual patient. It means integrating individual clinical expertise with the best available external clinical evidence from systematic research.* (Sackett et al. 1996: 71)

Since then the principles of evidence based practice have been adopted by many of the health professions and it is fair to say that evidence based practice is 'the integration of best research evidence with clinical experience and patient values' (Sackett et al. 2000: 1). The component parts of this definition will be considered in greater depth later on in the chapter.

Benefits of evidence based practice

The benefits of evidence based practice are basically that for the patient there would be less time wasted on inappropriate or ineffectual treatments with an enhanced consistency in care.

It was anticipated that the new approach to healthcare would elicit a greater understanding for patients of their investigations and treatments and this superior comprehension would promote increased confidence in both practitioners and the health system as a whole. From the practitioner's perspective it was suggested that through determining and incorporating the evidence they would be involved in identifying the most appropriate and effective care for their patients, which could then be audited. This active involvement would in turn enable practitioners to justify any changes to patient care that they felt necessary, thus strengthening professional accountability. It is important to remember that as a paramedic you are accountable for your actions (HPC 2008). Therefore it is important that you are aware of what constitutes best practice and how to implement it in your clinical work.

Evidence and quality

It was believed that implementation of evidence, in whatever appropriate form, would lead to a reduction in variation in health services through increasingly consistent decision making. A clear evidence base would also lend itself to the use of clearer quality measures such as audit, research, and quality assurance and enhancement, which would in turn strengthen the evidence base further, driving equitable and cost effective healthcare. All of these activities lead to further professionalisation of paramedic practice (Woollard 2009), hence appropriate implementation of evidence based practice can only serve to carry paramedic practice forward.

The origins and purpose of clinical governance and evidence based practice

The concept of clinical governance was introduced to the National Health Service (DH 1997) to enhance the management and monitoring of the quality of clinical care: evidence based practice being an integral part of the quality framework of clinical governance. Clinical governance required that care delivery be based on sound evidence that had proven to be effective clinically and also challenged practitioners to identify and improve poor practice.

Clinical governance brought ownership of the quality assurance activities into the NHS, thus quality became everyone's responsibility at individual, team and organisational levels. There are both professional and educational expectations that paramedics will incorporate the principles of clinical governance in their daily practice (QAA 2004; CoP 2008; Woollard 2009). Clinical governance comprises a number of key concepts and processes including (Sale 2005):

- patient and public involvement

- risk management

- clinical audit

- staffing and staff management

- education, training and continuing personal and professional development

- clinical effectiveness and use of clinical information to inform practice.

Evidence based practice is an integral part of clinical effectiveness which aims to ensure that practitioners do the right thing, in the right way and at the right time to the right patient (Royal College of Nursing 1996). This definition is applicable to all practitioners across the wide variety of healthcare settings. The combination of sound research knowledge, mature clinical decision making and involvement of the patient in the decision wherever possible will ensure that the 'rights' are achieved.

Development and continued refinement of the evidence base are informed by the National Institute for Health and Clinical Excellence (NICE) and National Service Frameworks (NSFs). NICE is the independent organisation responsible for providing national guidance on the promotion of good health and the prevention and treatment of ill health (NICE 2009). NSFs are used to promote national standards

Table 3.1 Examples of clinical guidelines relevant to paramedic practice

Document	Relevance to paramedic practice
NSF for Coronary Heart Disease (DH 2000)	Recommendations for: • multi-professional plans of management of people with suspected acute myocardial infarction • minimal time lapse for thrombolysis • an agreed service-wide protocol for the management of suspected acute myocardial infarction
Guidelines for Triage, Assessment, Investigation and Early Management of Head Injury in Infants, Children and Adults (NICE 2007)	Recommendations for: • collaborative planning for transfer of patients from hospital to neuro-centre • ambulance crews to be fully trained in use of Glasgow Coma Scale for adults and children • ambulance crews to be trained in the detection of non-accidental injuries

and guidelines wherever appropriate. Evidence from both sources can be seen to influence paramedic practice as highlighted in Table 3.1.

The purpose of clinical governance and related activities such as evidence based practice is to deliver the best quality of care that is possible within healthcare systems and organisations. Therefore evidence based practice should underpin all healthcare interventions including paramedic practice (QAA 2004). Using an evidence base makes it easier to include current best research evidence in healthcare decisions in order to promote clinical effectiveness.

The components of evidence based practice

The provision of high quality professional paramedic care is dependent upon up-to-date clinical knowledge and expertise (Clark 2006), both of which are vital components of evidence based practice. Changes in demographics, healthcare advances and technologies in the face of increasingly limited resources have necessitated a more rationalistic approach to care. It has become increasingly important to provide care that not only incorporates the best research evidence but is also clinically and financially effective, and takes into account patients' and professionals' expectations. The combinations of factors which contribute to evidence based practice are: research; clinical expertise; patient preference; and resources as shown in Figure 3.1.

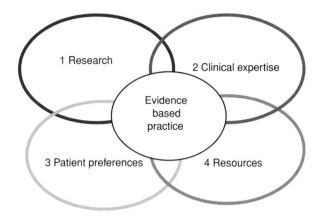

Figure 3.1 The components of evidence based practice

Research

Clinically relevant research that has been undertaken using sound methodology is accepted by most as the best evidence to guide practice (Sackett et al. 2000). It is fair to say however that robust evidence is not easily available for all aspects of paramedic practice and the time it will take for the profession to develop a strong evidence base may be considerable. It is suggested by Campeau (2008) that because paramedic science lacks the history of a professional presence such as medicine and the occupational research base of nursing it is therefore often thought of as a profession with a hybrid of knowledge and skills taken from other pre-established occupations. In order to establish their true professional identity paramedics need to develop their own research base, in the face of constantly changing practice. A number of research priorities for paramedics have been identified (Snooks et al. 2009), the main priority being the development of more relevant and meaningful performance measures other than response time, currently the single standard against which quality of the ambulance service is judged.

Whilst the paramedic profession strives to establish its own research and evidence base it is necessary for paramedics to use the best available evidence and Muir-Gray (1997) has attempted to aid that assessment of the strength of various types of evidence through the production of a hierarchy of evidence (see Table 3.2) which still stands today. The application of critical appraisal skills (Chapter 5) is vital for paramedics trying to discriminate between research evidence of varying calibres. Without these skills it is impossible to determine the quality of research evidence at any level of the hierarchy and findings from poor quality research may unwittingly be applied to paramedic practice with less favourable outcomes for the patient or the paramedic. This hierarchy of evidence, although well established, is not totally accepted by all practitioners as there is a sense that it excludes aspects of evidence drawn from clinical experience or some qualitative studies. This exclusion is felt by some to perpetuate the dominance of medicine and

Table 3.2 Hierarchy of evidence (Muir-Gray 1997: 61)

Strong evidence from at least one systematic review of multiple, well-designed randomised
    controlled trials (RCT)
Strong evidence from at least one properly designed RCT of appropriate size
Evidence from well-designed trials without randomisation, single group pre-post, cohort,
    time series or matched case control studies
Evidence from well-designed non-experimental studies from more than one centre or
    research group
Opinions of respected authorities, based clinical evidence, descriptive studies or reports of
    expert committees

pharmacological interventions above other healthcare professionals and their practices (Sale 2005). This domination is believed by some to prohibit the inclusion of intuitive knowledge (discussed in Chapter 2) which is much harder to explore, articulate or prove.

Clinical opinion and expertise

In order to achieve best outcomes research, wherever studies sit within the hierarchy, this knowledge needs to be combined with clinical expertise in order to make an informed decision about the appropriateness of any intervention. Many critics of the evidence based practice movement argue that it curtails individual clinical judgement. McSherry et al. (2002) however suggest that when incorporated correctly professional opinion is an integral part of evidence based practice. Evidence cannot replace clinical judgement; rather, when applied appropriately it can enhance that judgement. Equally, clinical judgement is required in order to appraise the research and to determine its relevance and weight in relation to individual cases. Paramedics make clinical judgements as part of their daily practice and they are encouraged to acknowledge that research knowledge has limitations and professional judgement is paramount, at the same time recognising their own limitations and practice within those (QAA 2004).

Clinical expertise and opinion are increasingly important in paramedic practice with the evolution of the advanced paramedic practitioner (APP) role. There is a recognised need for these practitioners to make sound judgements when faced with extra-ordinary clinical situations. It is acknowledged that paramedics' clinical decision making about best and most appropriate treatment is complex and multi-faceted (Porter et al. 2007). Paramedics need to be able to work with their patients in order to find practical and often unique solutions to the problems they encounter in practice. This is in part achieved by their required ability to appraise the available evidence in an attempt to determine the potential effects of their interventions or omissions of care in order to make their professional judgements (QAA 2004).

Patient preferences

Working within guidelines and using their own clinical judgement, paramedics still have to gain information from patients to enable the best informed decision about treatments. Patient preference and opinions about care and treatment options are becoming increasingly important in the evidence based practice debate with better access to healthcare information and the advent of expert patients and patient advocacy services. Patient opinions can no longer be ignored as they were in the past when healthcare tended to be far more paternalistic; ideally there should be shared decision making between patients and healthcare professionals.

Ultimately patient preference can significantly influence paramedic practice as it is the patient alone who can make the decision not to be taken to hospital as far as they are deemed to have the mental capacity to make that decision (Porter et al. 2007). Without patient concordance nothing will work! Patients may not like a certain drug, dressing or intervention or may not wish to leave their home.

Resources

All healthcare is provided within an increasingly restrictive budget, therefore resources are central to all decision making. Care options may therefore be determined by resource allocation. Whilst it has been proven that for some patients transport to hospital by air ambulance significantly improves patient survival, by reducing time to reach a healthcare facility to receive definitive treatment (Moga and Harstall 2009). It is not however viable economically to establish air ambulance services everywhere.

Sources of evidence

The evidence base for unscheduled urgent care and paramedic practice is developing and paramedics need to be aware of the research that has informed the service to date. Critical evaluative skills are vital to enable paramedics to make an informed decision about the intervention under examination. There are a number of sources of evidence which can be drawn upon to inform practice. Each type of evidence has strengths and weaknesses as identified in Table 3.3.

Strengthening the evidence base for paramedic practice

A review of the research literature related to paramedic practice concluded that there is limited high quality evidence against which principal actions of paramedic practice could be validated (Ball 2005). There is an expectation that paramedics will contribute to the developing evidence base for unscheduled urgent care, by evaluating critically the literature, implementing findings into their practice where

Table 3.3 Strengths and weaknesses of different sources of evidence

Source of evidence	Strengths of evidence source	Weaknesses of evidence source
Books	Reliable for information that does not change e.g. anatomy and physiology	Date very quickly therefore not reliable source for current or dynamic evidence relating to practice
Research articles	More current information	Articles may refer to dated data Research may not be robust, ethical
Evidence based journals	Present précis of robust research studies, aids rapid decision making about inclusion or exclusion of studies	May lack some of the finite detail so better to read whole article if you can
Systematic reviews e.g. Cochrane Database of Abstracts of Reviews of Effect (DARE)	Well-defined methodology results in systematic reviews constituting strong evidence within hierarchy	Review may be dated before/shortly after completion Potential selection bias
Internet	Provides access to the most current information Good quality professional sites provide clinically relevant research e.g. College of Paramedics, Department of Health	Internet is not regulated for quality of content therefore the website may be disreputable and the information unreliable Quality of a website can be judged using quality indicators identified in the Health on the Net Foundation code (2002)
Practice documents such as polices, clinical guidelines, algorithms, integrated pathways (JRCALC, NICE, NSFs)	Bring together best evidence, clinical expertise, multi-professional collaboration and user/patient opinions Can change clinical practice to improve patient outcomes	May be perceived as: unrealistic, irrelevant, restrictive, challenging to clinical autonomy May be gaps in evidence so documents incomplete

Table 3.4 Developing sources of paramedic evidence

Type of paramedic evidence	Authors/collators/sources
Précis of quality emergency/paramedic research Practice guidelines	Pre-hospital evidence based protocol project (Canada – Jensen et al. 2009) Joint Royal Colleges Ambulance Liaison Committee (JRCALC) (2009) *Emergency Medicine Journal*
Database of studies relevant to emergency and urgent care (including Cochrane, DARE)	NHS evidence website
Key findings from relevant research studies and reviews	Emergency Service Current Awareness Updates (published by the National Ambulance Research Steering Group)

appropriate, and contributing to the development of evidence based guidelines and protocols (QAA 2004; Woollard 2009). Paramedic groups are actively seeking to address this in a number of ways as identified in Table 3.4.

Barriers to evidence based practice

Rigorous evaluation of implementation strategies highlight that even in areas where the evidence is indisputable compliance to best practice is often sub-optimal (van Achterberg et al. 2008). It is therefore apparent that a number of barriers to the implementation of best evidence based practice persist. Some of these barriers are presented in Table 3.5.

Implementing evidence based practice

Evidence based practice, when done properly, is a cyclical process. There are clear steps involved in the implementation of evidence based practice as illustrated in Figure 3.2.

Step 1: Identify a problem in practice

Often pursuit of the best available evidence arises from a practitioner's hunch that an intervention could or should be changed or improved. For example, why are we transporting dying patients to hospital when they want to remain at home? At this point it is useful to discuss your ideas with colleagues, preferably with a multi-disciplinary focus to increase the breadth of the discussion. From these discussions it is necessary to formulate a question in order to guide the literature searching and reviewing: this question and subsequent exploration of the literature will enable you to determine the gap between your current practice and best practice. When forming a question it is important to be focussed and clear to ensure that the

Table 3.5 Barriers to evidence based practice

Identified barrier	Consequence of barrier	Possible solution
No research available on topic or research evidence available is poor quality	No existing stringent evidence base	Need to seek expert clinical opinion and start to develop the evidence base through appropriate research methods
Best evidence being neither accessible nor comprehensible	Practitioners unable to access evidence therefore cannot build evidence base	May need assistance of proficient researcher/ librarian to access and translate research into comprehensible terms
Practitioners lack time to access and appraise evidence	Practitioners are therefore unable to formulate questions, access, and critique or identify the evidence base	Allocation of protected time for practitioners involved in evidence based projects.
Practitioners lack critical appraisal skills		Appropriate training in critical appraisal skills
Research not perceived as applicable to practice	Practitioners are reluctant to accept or apply the evidence	Communication with practitioners to raise awareness of applicability of research
		Possible involvement of a change champion or respected clinical expert.
Poor communication of either the need for change or the processes involved in the implementation	Practitioners do not see the need for the proposed change or do not feel involved in the process, have no ownership of the change so are reluctant to adapt their practice to fit the change	Improved two way communication
		Facilitation of meetings to aid involvement and sense of ownership
Resistance to change due to variety of reasons that include: • Lack of understanding of process or implications • Lack of trust • Fear, anxiety or uncertainty • Tradition • Sense of loss • Lack necessary skills	Practitioners will not adopt change	Improved two way communications to aid expression and understanding of reasons for resistance Acknowledgement of these reasons and feelings Supportive exploration and negotiation of ways forward Appropriate training to attend to any skills deficit

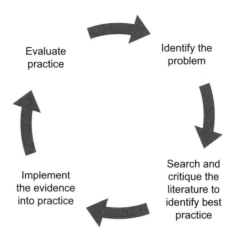

Figure 3.2 Stages involved in evidence based practice

question is relevant and that it will yield the information required. There are three or four points to be considered in a question:

1   the patient

2   the intervention

3   comparative interventions (optional)

4   the outcome.

For all four points it is vital to be focussed and precise. The question needs to be sufficiently specific to highlight all potential areas for that patient or the patient group under consideration.

For example, you may be a paramedic who has recently moved employers. Since changing jobs you notice that a significantly greater amount of your time is being spent transferring dying patients from home to hospital than in your previous job. Patients are being admitted for management of pain and other symptoms that general practitioners (GPs) have been unable to control. You start to think what the differences might be and remember that in your previous job the GPs had 24-hour access to telephone support and medical management advice from a specialist palliative care team. Through discussion with colleagues it becomes apparent that this service does not exist in your new area. This leads you and your colleagues to ask the question:

> Does access to 24-hour specialist palliative care support and advice (intervention) result in fewer dying patients (patient) being admitted to hospital end of life management (outcome)?

Step 2: Search and appraise the literature

It is necessary to undertake a comprehensive literature search and review before attempting to change practice in order to ensure that proposed change is the right change and that it is informed by available evidence. So, having determined your question the next stage is to search the literature. This activity is primarily concerned with searching clinically relevant databases such as MEDLINE, EMBASE, CINAHL, PsycInfo and Cochrane to obtain relevant research evidence that will potentially inform your practice. Returning to your question will help you decide what key search terms you should use. Help from a librarian is invaluable for a novice searcher as each database has its own peculiarities such as filters, truncations with which you will eventually become familiar. Searching and appraising the literature is discussed in Chapter 5 but in order to answer the question above key search terms would be words such as:

> *specialist palliative care, dying patients, community care, GP knowledge, GP practice, pain and symptom management, end of life care, hospital admission, prevention.*

Using inclusion and exclusion criteria as discussed later you decide which literature you are going to review. You then read and critically appraise the literature and pull out the main findings and recommendations as discussed in Chapter 5. Some findings lend themselves to straightforward implementation through development of algorithms, guidelines, care pathways or protocols, whereas other changes may be more abstract and difficult to determine. In this example it is likely that the literature will suggest (as your previous practice will confirm) that GPs and community nursing teams need to have good knowledge of general palliative care and access to 24-hour specialist palliative care support.

Step 3: Implement your findings from the literature review

Having appraised the literature, key findings will emerge and the next step in the evidence based practice process is to look at ways of implementing these findings into your practice. This is fraught with challenges and barriers. Some of the key principles of getting the evidence into practice relate to the long-established processes involved in the leadership and management of change. There are a number of comprehensive books that cover this topic, for instance Broome (1998), Jasper and Juma (2005) and Hartley and Bennington (2010). You are recommended to read at least one before embarking on the introduction of new practice into your area, and it always worth gaining the support of a respected clinical expert to motivate and communicate with colleagues.

The most important things to remember when trying to change practice are to communicate the need for change effectively at all levels across the organisation, to get people to agree to the need for change and to be involved in the change. It takes time and energy to support the introduction of new practice and to help colleagues adopt that practice.

Step 4: Evaluate the impact of the implementation

After an allotted time it is necessary to evaluate the change in order to see if it has achieved its aim, such as reducing the number of transfers of dying patients from home to hospital because of poor pain control. If the change has been ineffectual it is necessary to review practice again and consider alternative, evidence based interventions. The effects of the implementation needs to be evaluated against predetermined outcome measures. It is good practice to identify evaluation methods at the beginning of the evidence based project along with all the other strategies that are going to be involved throughout. The findings from the evaluation should be reported upon and disseminated amongst all who have been involved in or affected by the change.

Conclusion

Evidence based practice, the 'integration of best research evidence with clinical experience and patient values' (Sackett et al. 2000: 1), is an integral component of clinical governance which was introduced to counteract deficits in care in order to improve the quality of care and increase public confidence in the National Health Service. Evidence based practice enables practitioners to provide clinically and cost effective care to an ever-increasing population in a time of increased technology and scarce resources. Evidence can be rated according to an established hierarchy of evidence but other contextual evidence and information needs to be taken into account including patient preference, clinical expertise and opinion, and resource implications. In order to determine the evidence base it is necessary to start with clear, focussed questions relating to patient or client needs, interventions or outcomes. Proven implementation strategies and effective communication need to be applied in order to effect introduction of new clinical practices in light of the emerging evidence base. Failure to attend to this will result in resistance to change and the failure to move practice forward. Stringent evaluation is necessary to assess whether or not the implementation of the evidence base has resulted in improved outcomes of care, or service. If not, then it is necessary to go back to the drawing board to rediscover just what is best evidence and how it might be most effectively implemented into paramedic practice.

References

Ball, L. (2005) Setting the scene for the paramedic in primary care: a review of the literature. *Emergency Medicine Journal* 22: 896–900.

Broome, A. (1998) *Managing Change* (2nd edn). Basingstoke: Macmillan.

Campeau, A. (2008) Why paramedics require 'theories of practice'. *Journal of Emergency Primary Care* 6(2): 1–7.

Clark, T. (2006) Foreword. In: Fisher, J.D., Brown, S.N. and Cooke, M.W. (eds) *UK Ambulance Service Clinical Practice Guidelines*. London: JRCALC and Ambulance Service Association.

College of Paramedics/British Paramedic Association (2008) *Paramedic Curriculum Guidance and Competence Framework* (2nd edn). Derby: College of Paramedics.

Department of Health (1997) *The New NHS: Modern, Dependable*. London: DH.

Department of Health (1998) *A First Class Service: Quality in the New NHS*. London: DH.
Department of Health (2000) *National Service Framework for Coronary Heart Disease*. Available
    at: http://www.dh.gov.uk/prod_consum_dh/groups/dh_digitalassets/@dh/@en/
    documents/digitalasset/dh_4057526.pdf [accessed 17 March 2011].
Hartley, J. and Bennington, J. (2010) *Leadership for Healthcare*. Bristol: Policy Press.
Health Professions Council (2008) *Standards of Conduct, Performance and Ethics*. London:
    HPA. Available at: www.hpc-uk.org [accessed 23 August 2009].
Jasper, M. and Juma, M. (eds) (2005) *Effective Healthcare Leadership*. Oxford: Blackwell
    Publishing.
Jensen, J., Petrie, D., Cain, E. and Travers, A. (2009) The Canadian prehospital evidence
    based protocols project: knowledge translation in emergency medical services care.
    Academic Emergency Medicine 16: 668–673.
Joint Royal Colleges Ambulance Liaison Committee (2009) *Guidelines*. Available at:
    http://www.jrcalc.org.uk/ [accessed 17 March 2011].
McSherry, R., Simmons, M. and Abbott, P. (2002) An introduction to evidence-informed
    nursing. In: McSherry, R., Simmons, M. and Abbott, P. (eds) *Evidence-Informed Nursing: A
    Guide for Clinical Nurses*. London: Routledge.
Moga, C. and Harstall, C. (2009) *Air Ambulance Transportation with Capabilities to Provide
    Advanced Life Support*. Database of Abstracts of Reviews of Effects. Available at: http://
    www.crd.york.ac.uk/CMS2Web/ShowRecord.asp?LinkFrom=OAI&ID=12008105051
    [accessed 19 February].
Muir-Gray, J.A. (1997) *Evidence Based Healthcare: How to Make Health Policy and Management
    Decisions*. London: Churchill Livingstone.
National Institute for Health and Clinical Excellence (2007) *Guidelines for Triage, Assessment,
    Investigation and Early Management of Head Injury in Infants, Children and Adults*. Available
    at: http://guidance.nice.org.uk/CG56 [accessed 19 February 2011].
National Institute for Health and Clinical Excellence (2009) *About NICE*. Available at:
    http://www.nice.org.uk/aboutnice/ [accessed 19 February 2011].
Porter, A., Snooks, H., Youren, A. et al. (2007) Should I stay or should I go? Deciding whether
    to go to hospital after a 999 call. *Journal of Health Services Research and Policy* 12(Suppl. 1):
    32–38.
Quality Assurance Agency for Higher Education (2004) *Paramedic Science, Benchmark
    Statement: Health Care Programmes Phase 2*. Gloucester: QAA.
Royal College of Nursing (1996) *What is Clinical Effectiveness?* London: RCN.
Sackett, D.L., Richardson, W.S., Rosenberg, W. and Haynes, R.B. (1996) *Evidence-based
    Medicine: How to Practise and Teach EBM*. New York: Churchill Livingstone.
Sackett, D.L., Richardson, W.S., Rosenberg, W. and Haynes, R.B. (2000) *Evidence-based
    Medicine: How to Practice and Teach EBM* (2nd edn). Edinburgh: Churchill Livingstone.
Sale, D. (2005) *Understanding Clinical Governance and Quality Assurance: Making it Happen*.
    Basingstoke: Palgrave Macmillan.
Snooks, H., Evans, A., Wells, B. et al. (2009) What are the highest priorities for research in
    emergency prehospital care? *Emergency Medicine Journal* 26(8): 549–550.
van Achterberg, T., Schoonhoven, L. and Grol, R. (2008) Nursing implementation science:
    how evidence based nursing requires evidence based implementation. *Journal of Nursing
    Scholarship* 40(4): 302–310.
Woollard, M. (2009) Professionalism in UK paramedic practice. *Journal of Emergency Primary
    Health Care* 7(4): article 990391.

Useful evidence based practice websites/databases

Bandolier http://www.medicine.ox.ac.uk/bandolier/
Best bets http://www.bestbets.org/

Centre for Evidence Based Medicine www.cebm.net/index.aspx?o=1001
Centre for Reviews and Dissemination www.york.ac.uk/inst/crd/index.htm
Cochrane Centre http://www.cochrane.co.uk/en/index.html
College of Paramedics https://www.collegeofparamedics.co.uk/home/
Critical Skills Appraisal Programme www.phru.nhs.uk/Pages/PHD/CASP.htm
Joanna Briggs Institute www.joannabriggs.edu.au/about/home.php
Joint Royal Colleges Ambulance Liaison Committee http://jrcalc.org.uk/
NHS Evidence – emergency and urgent care http://www.library.nhs.uk/Emergency/
Scottish Intercollegiate Guidelines Network www.sign.ac.uk/index.html

4 Conducting ethical research in paramedic practice

Pauline Griffiths

Learning outcomes for the chapter
By the end of this chapter the reader should be able to:

1   Understand the function of research ethics committees

2   Describe what research governance is

3   Understand why individual autonomy and rights to self-determination must underpin ethical research activity

4   Consider the principle of non-maleficence(doing no harm) during research studies

Keywords
autonomy
informed consent
non maleficence
research governance

Introduction

Ensuring that ethical research conduct is maintained throughout all stages of the research process is a vital consideration for those undertaking research. When reading research papers, an essential component of the evaluation of research is being able to critique, in an informed manner, the ethical approach that a study has taken (PHRU 2007). The paramedic has also a responsibility to ensure that researchers act in an ethically appropriate manner when they access patients, carers or colleagues for whom the paramedic holds a duty of care (Griffiths 2006). Researchers have a legal, a moral and, as is the case with the researcher who is also a registered paramedic, a professional responsibility to ensure that the rights of research participants are protected. This chapter provides a general overview to research ethics applicable to paramedic research practice drawing on core ethical concepts.

What will paramedics research?

Paramedic research may help explore the experiences of patients, carers or health-care staff and students, or the researcher may interrogate data held related to individuals or to client groups. The researcher has a responsibility to conduct research that is undertaken in a suitably stringent manner and to deliver findings that are relevant and satisfy the 'so-what' criteria:

- Will the research findings lead to advances in paramedic practice or education?
- Is there a potential for the research findings to improve patient care?

If the research cannot satisfy these requirements then we can be justified in asking why it is being done and why participants' time is being wasted. Research governance is the term that captures these expectations of worthwhile and ethically appropriate empirical investigation.

Research governance

Research governance provides regulations, principles and standards of good practice to ensure that research studies are suitably planned and demonstrate ethical appropriateness. Paramedic research will often involve National Health Service patients or their data and an NHS Research Ethics Committee (REC) must sanction research proposals when NHS patients, their tissue, data or information related to their relatives, NHS staff or NHS premises are involved (DH England 2005; Department of Health, Social Services and Public Safety (Northern Ireland) 2002); Scottish Executive Health Department 2006; Welsh Assembly Government 2002). (See Figure 4.1)

Box 4.1 is an example of a real research study which we have included to demonstrate key ethical aspects of research in practice.

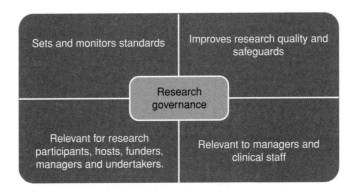

Figure 4.1 Research governance (adapted from DH 2005)

Box 4.1 Research governance in action

Pre-hospital randomised assessment of a mechanical compression device in cardiac arrest (PaRAMeDIC) trial protocol (Perkins et al. 2010)

This paper describes a study that will seek to compare short- and long-term patient outcomes following cardiac arrest using two different approaches to chest compressions: a) mechanical compression device and b) standard manual chest compression. 4000 participants will be included and selected randomly to one of the two groups. Exclusion criteria include being less than 18 years of age, being pregnant, or suffering a traumatic cardiac arrest.

By definition consent cannot be gained; however, the Local Research Ethics Committee has agreed a waiver of consent. Participants who survive will be asked for their consent during the follow-up phase.

The authors note that 'The trial is registered on the International Standard Randomised Controlled Trial Registry (ISRCTN08233942)'. It will be carried out in accordance with the Medical Research Council (MRC) Good Clinical Practice Guidelines [13], applicable UK legislation and the Standard Operating Procedures of the Warwick Clinical Trials Unit. The sponsor organisation for the trial is the University of Warwick. The trial is funded by the National Institute for Health Research (NIHR) Health Technology Assessment (HTA) Programme [14] and is a collaboration between the Universities of Warwick, Coventry, Leeds, Southampton and Surrey and the West Midlands, Scottish and Welsh NHS Ambulance Services' (p. 2).

Research governance as applied to research

The research study described in Box 4.1 is a complex one especially in terms of the ethics of the study and its research governance. In Figure 4.1 core research governance responsibilities are noted; from this we can see that this study (as described) is well thought out and demonstrates good research practice:

1   The research approach demonstrates adherence and accordance with the research governance requirements of England, Wales and Scotland and the authors have detailed the wide-ranging scrutiny this research study has been exposed to.

2   Such complex research projects require close scrutiny, but equally important is that research quality and safeguards can be enhanced by the research governance precedents set by such studies. Importantly, the authors note that manufacturers of the device played no part in the study design, only providing training to its users. This ensures that undue pressure from the manufacturers for a positive result will not be possible.

3   Paramedics and their managers involved in the study can be assured that the study has been well designed and does not pose a risk to their patients or to their professional integrity.

4 If this study indicates that there are better outcomes using this device then its increased use could improve patient mortality and morbidity. Or if the study disproves its effectiveness practitioners and researchers can work towards developing other modes and methods of delivering effective external cardiac massage.

Research participants and hosts of research can be assured that this study has undergone close research governance scrutiny and that monitoring of its undertaking will serve the good of society. To enable this judgement to be made the researchers were required to develop a comprehensive research proposal.

Research proposals

Research proposals outline the planned conduct of the study and offer evidence that the research will be conducted appropriately and in an ethically responsible manner. The preparation of a comprehensive research proposal is time well spent and helps the researcher consider fully the intended research approach. There is now a single system for applying for ethical approval for health and social care/community care research in the UK called the Integrated Research Application System (IRAS) that has expedited this process. Whereas multisite studies used to require approval from all the RECs within the study's range, happily now a coordinated system for gaining NHS permissions has been developed (IRAS 2009). This includes a 'passport' for researchers who are non-NHS staff, and whose research is likely to impact on patient care, to obtain an NHS Honorary Contract that is transferable between research sites (UK Clinical Research Collaboration (UKCRC) 2009).

Other forms of independent ethical review may be required if the intended participants are students or academic staff through a University Research Ethics Committee. NHS Ambulance Trusts are likely to have their own research ethics committee at which research proposals involving Trust staff and premises, patients or patient information will be reviewed. Consideration of research conduct will require certain core ethical principles to be addressed; these principles are discussed next.

Ethical research

Whilst individual rights have been infringed over the centuries in the name of research it was the atrocities perpetuated under the guise of medical research by the Nazi regime during the Second World War that caused worldwide revulsion. Following this shameful misuse (and often death) of unwilling research subjects the Nuremberg Code of ethical requirements for human biomedical experimentation was developed in 1949. The medical profession endorsed this initiative within the Declaration of Helsinki with the Code being revised frequently since then and most recently in 2008 (World Medical Association 2008). All professional codes of ethical research practice draw on this guidance. The College of Paramedics (CoM) does not offer specific written guidance on research ethics at present but the College's research and audit committee members can offer individual guidance and will peer-review research proposals prior to submission to ethics committees.

Despite the Declaration of Helsinki the abuse of research subjects can still occur. One notorious example is 'The Tuskegee Syphilis Trial' (see Box 4.2).

Box 4.2 The Tuskegee Syphilis Trial

The Tuskegee Syphilis Trial (Centers Disease Control and Protection 2009)

This study sought to understand the long-term effects of syphilis on a group of African-American men over a 40-year period. When this study commenced in 1932 treatments for syphilis were often potentially toxic, and thus dangerous to the patient, and so comparing treatment with non-treatment was ethically acceptable.

From 1947 onwards penicillin, which is a cure for syphilis, was readily available but this treatment was not offered to the subjects in this experiment, nor were they told of this option. The withholding of treatment resulted in these men moving to the tertiary phase of the disease when widespread tumour-like masses called *gummas* damage the heart and blood vessels (cardiovascular syphilis) and the brain (neuro-syphilis) causing them to experience a miserable quality of life and an early death.

The moral wrongness of this project was further compounded by the infection of the men's wives with syphilis and the birth of children with congenital syphilis that can cause blindness from birth and learning difficulties.

Although we can look back and see how ethically inappropriate this behaviour was, it must be remembered that doctors, nurses and other healthcare workers were involved with this study and no concern was raised until the 1970s. What this shocking example demonstrates is that the vigilance as to the moral conduct of researchers and the ethical appropriateness of a study cannot be overestimated and that seeking knowledge must never compromise human rights: for informed consent is 'the heart of ethical research' (DH 2005: 11). Respecting research participants' dignity, rights, safety and wellbeing are the primary concerns of researchers (DH 2005). The ethical principles of autonomy and non-maleficence, a responsibility not to cause harm, offer overarching principles to consider the ethical concepts that should inform research and are discussed next.

Autonomy

Gillon (1986: 60) defines autonomy as being 'the capacity to think, decide, and act on the basis of such thought and decision freely and independently and without let or hindrance'. This principle is enshrined in the common law of the four countries of the United Kingdom and by other democratic countries across the world. Rights to personal autonomy were further enhanced in the UK following the passing in 1998 of the Human Rights Act.

An ethical consideration of autonomy related to research studies gives us six key ethical and legal concepts to consider: consent and informed consent; privacy and confidentiality; veracity (truth telling) and fidelity (building of trust). These ethical principles are discussed next.

Consent and informed consent

Consent is a common law rather than a statute law, which means that understanding of this legal concept has developed over the years by precedent case law, rather than by formal legislation being enacted. Consent in common law relates to a clear permission, implied or expressed, to allow one person to touch another person or to allow them to use personal information (Mason and McCall Smith 1994). The seminal statement of this concept was delivered in a US court ruling by Judge Cardozo in 1934 who stated that:

> *Every human being of adult years and sound mind has a right to determine what shall be done with his own body: and a surgeon who performs an operation without the patient's consent commits an assault.* (cited in Mason and McCall Smith 1994: 219)

Therefore to touch another person without their consent constitutes an assault or a battery to the person, dealt with in either the civil or the criminal courts dependent on the severity of the battery (Mason and McCall Smith 1994). This is why the Health Professions Council (HPC 2008) requires that paramedics seek the patient's consent before touching them or giving them treatments. It is important to remember that if the patient is an adult (i.e. over 18 years of age) no one can give consent for them unless a designated decision maker has been appointed under the Mental Capacity Act 2005 (Griffith and Tengnah 2010).

In those cases where the adult patient lacks mental capacity to provide consent, such as when unconscious, the paramedic then acts in the patient's best interests to save life or prevent serious injury. This is a form of presumed consent in a situation of necessity. In the case of children their parents or guardians give consent but parents or guardians have no legal right to give or to withhold consent if this would cause the child harm. Paramedics may have to treat a seriously ill child even if the parents object. Clearly, however, the legal acceptance of unconsented treatment does not apply when seeking consent from research participants:

> *Participation by competent individuals as subjects in medical research must be voluntary. Although it may be appropriate to consult family members or community leaders, no competent individual may be enrolled in a research study unless he or she freely agrees.* (WMA 2008: s. 22)

Gaining consent from would-be research participants is a fundamental consideration within an ethical research process. The researcher must be aware of and respect the law related to consent and professional guidance. The Nuremberg Code notes at section 1 that:

> *The duty and responsibility for ascertaining the quality of the consent rests upon each individual who initiates, directs or engages in the experiment. It is a personal duty and responsibility which may not be delegated to another with impunity.* (cited by National Institute of Health 2010: 1)

The responsibility and accountability of the researcher, especially the designated Chief Investigator, is therefore a core element of research governance. This person must ensure that the participants know that they are involved in a research study and that they are fully aware of the risks and benefits of being involved. Consent must be informed consent. The gaining of informed consent needs special consideration when a paramedic is acting in a dual role as both a practitioner and a researcher. If I collect data whilst providing care then express consent is needed from the patient to both the care intervention and to the collection of research data. If I am however treating a patient, and whilst doing so I seek consent to collect data, might this have the potential for being coercive as I am in a powerful position in relation to the patient? The patient may not like to refuse consent to participate in the study as they could worry that this refusal might affect their treatment in a negative manner (Winch et al. 2008). Researchers must ask of themselves such questions and offer solutions that have been considered ethically. Research committees, and readers of their subsequent papers, most certainly will expect well-thought-out answers. Consider the example in Box 4.3.

Box 4.3 Gaining consent (1)

Safety of paramedics with extended skills (Mason et al. 2008)

Mason and colleagues sought to evaluate the safety of clinical decisions made by extended-role paramedic practitioners (PP) when managing minor acute illness and injury among older people in their homes and seeking to avoid, when suitable, unnecessary transfer to the emergency department (ED). The study design was a cluster-randomised controlled trial ($n = 2025$). Some patients were treated with the new PP intervention and some the standard practice outcomes. Their outcomes were then compared using their clinical records. Participants were selected following a call to the Emergency Medical Services control room with a condition eligible for PP assessment. During 'intervention weeks' a PP provided care and during 'control weeks' patients were transferred to the ED. Findings indicate that the PP intervention groups were at least as safe as those receiving standard care.

Ethical approach

Patients had given written consent to follow-up following face-to-face contact. Local research ethics approval from the North Sheffield Research Ethics Committee had been obtained.

When consent cannot be achieved at the time of data collection the researcher can seek retrospective or delayed consent and the participant is approached when they have regained the mental or physical capacity to provide consent (Long 2007). Provided that the data collection does not cause risk to the participant and there is likely to be benefit from the study's findings then data could be collected subject to REC approval (Long 2007). This was also the case in the research study discussed earlier (Box 4.1). The assumption is that agreement will be forthcoming and consent is presumed, that is, the participant would have given consent had they had the mental capacity. However, if when approached the patient then should refuse to give retrospective consent any data collected would have to be destroyed.

In the study discussed in Box 4.3 paramedics treated patients but these patients were also subjects in a randomised controlled trial. Questions to ask are:

- Did the patients realise during treatment they were part of a research study?

- They consented to receiving care from a paramedic but they did not consent to being a research subject. Was this the right course of action?

- Did they give informed consent at the time of their treatment and was consent to collect follow up data collection sufficient?

The conditions for informed consent are detailed in Figure 4.2.

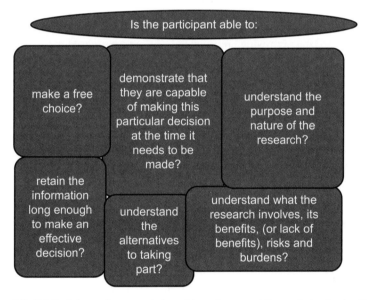

Figure 4.2 Gaining informed consent (adapted from Integrated Research Application System 2009)

On-going consent

Informed consent for treatment in paramedic practice is often related to immediate treatment whereas for research projects it is generally a prospective agreement, which brings its own concerns related to the gaining of on-going consent in those studies that require frequent contact. During overt participant observation during an ethnographic study of a medical assessment unit I became well known to all health staff on the unit and in many ways part of the team (Griffiths 2011). People became so relaxed with my presence that they spoke unguardedly. Whilst this often provided interesting data I was required to remind them frequently that I was a researcher and to ask if individuals were happy for me to add their comments to my field notes: not to do so would have been a form of deception. See Figure 4.2.

Using covert methods

Gaining data using covert (hidden) methods is increasingly being seen as ethically inappropriate and for most research studies covert methods would not be used. Johnson (2007) argues however that the use of covert methods may be ethically justifiable if topics cannot be researched by any other approach and findings would be in the public good. John Brewer, an ethnographer, wished to study former members of the British Union of Fascists and engaged in covert data collection: not without a degree of high risk to himself (Brewer 2000). The ethical justification for this covert data collection undertaken was a utilitarian argument (a belief that the moral worth of an action is judged by its ability to bring pleasure or benefit). This extreme right-wing group would not have permitted data collection if asked and Brewer argues that a greater good was served to society by the enhanced understanding of the group that his findings permitted.

Remaining critical

It is difficult for authors to capture all of the detail of a study in a published paper due to word constraints. Nonetheless a research paper that raises queries in the reader's mind as to its ethical conduct can be critiqued for not making the ethical approach clear. As the Tuskegee study shows we must guard against complacence: inappropriate ethical conduct risks participants suffering harm and we must always raise ethical challenges. Providing information and the signing of a consent form are strategies to gain informed consent.

Information literature and the consent form

Most research participants will be asked to sign a written consent form that records their agreement to be involved in the research study. Prior to signing the consent form the participant must be given information about the study, ideally in an easily understood written form or in some other suitable format, such as using pictures when approaching children or those who cannot read. This information will explain how involvement in the study will affect the participant including the demands on their time and details of the risks and benefits they face. Often there will be no measurable benefit for the participant other than the contribution that the study's findings will make to the advancement of knowledge. It must be noted clearly in all information provided, including the consent form, that the participant can withdraw their consent at any time with no negative repercussions. Consent must be given freely and the researcher must make it clear that no coercion will be or was used to gain agreement. This is summarised in Figure 4.3.

Minimum information on a research consent form

1 **Title of Project**
2 **Name of Researcher**
3 **Confirmation that the participant:**
   - has read and understand a dated study information sheet
   - has had the opportunity to consider the information, ask questions and have had these answered satisfactorily
   - understands that participation is voluntary and that they are free to withdraw at any time without giving any reason, without their healthcare or legal rights being affected
   - agrees to take part in the study
4 **Signatures and names written in capital letters of the participant and the researcher**
5 **Date that the consent was signed**
6 **Acknowledgment that the participant and the researcher will retain copies of the consent form**

Figure 4.3 Basic information on a consent form

In the study outlined in Box 4.4 we see that Cox et al. (2006) gained REC approval for the study, full information was given to participants, signed consent was obtained from all participants, and measures to ensure confidentiality were in place. This study, from the content of the published paper, was undertaken in a suitable manner as regards ethical research conduct.

An area of ethical consideration where the gaining of informed consent is more complex is when the researcher is seeking to access vulnerable groups.

Box 4.4 Gaining Consent (2)

Paramedics' perceptions of their role in providing pre-hospital thrombolytic treatment: qualitative study (Cox et al. 2006)

Cox and colleagues undertook a qualitative study using focus groups to gain understanding of paramedics' perceptions of providing thrombolytic treatment in the pre-hospital setting.

Twenty paramedics were included. Permission to undertake the study had been given by the local REC and the ambulance trust. Participants were asked if they would take part in the study directly whilst attending a training day. Detailed information sheets were provided and participants signed consent forms that noted their agreement to be part of the study and to the focus group to be audio-recorded and then transcribed using identifying numbers rather than names to ensure confidentiality.

Vulnerable groups

Enormous care must be taken when seeking to access vulnerable groups such as children and young people, the recently bereaved and those with mental health problems.

Children and young people

Children and young people are consumers of health and social care and research that seeks to understand their experiences and to improve care delivery is worthwhile. However, children and young people present a particular problem as to the appropriate way to gain consent. There must be a negligible risk of the child suffering harm if the research is non-therapeutic, and if the research involves therapeutic interventions the likely benefits must outweigh possible risks to the child (DH 2005).

There is no specific legislation related to children's and young people's involvement in research so we draw on the law on consent as it relates to medical treatment (Long 2007). The overriding legal principle is that the child's or young person's welfare must be considered paramount and the researcher is unlikely (but it is not impossible) to include an under-16-year-old in a study unless the parents agreed. Griffith and Tengnah (2010) discuss how the 16–18-year-old is assumed to have capacity to consent but sometimes considered not to have capacity should they, for instance, refuse treatment that is required to be undertaken in their best interest.

Pregnant women

When involving pregnant women in research studies concern as to the safety and wellbeing of the woman and the foetus must be evidenced. This leads to pregnant women being excluded from research studies, as was noted in the research discussed earlier into mechanical pressure devices used during cardiac arrest (Perkins et al. 2010). No reason for non-inclusion was given. This is often the case as the ability to define with complete confidence that there is no risk to the pregnant woman, or to the foetus, is very difficult, and RECs are particularly stringent on this issue. Researchers then often simply avoid recruiting pregnant women unless their inclusion in the sample is essential. This leads to pregnant women often being disadvantaged and being left at increased risk. Goldkind et al. (2010), for instance, noted that the global H1N1 influenza pandemic was affecting pregnant women disproportionately as they were excluded from drug trials related to vaccine development.

> Ironically, the effort to protect the fetus from research-related risks by excluding pregnant women from research places both women and their fetuses at greater risk from unstudied clinical interventions and may also result in a dearth of therapeutic options specifically developed for pregnant women. (Goldkind et al. 2010: 2243)

In-depth guidance regarding research involving children and young people or pregnant women is provided by the Department of Health (2005) and the Medical Research Council (MRC 2009). If you are critiquing a paper, or preparing to undertake research involving these groups, you are strongly advised to read these documents carefully.

The bereaved

Vulnerable groups can include the bereaved and the researcher must exercise special thoughtfulness. For instance, a paramedic researcher may wish to interview parents who have experienced sudden infant death syndrome seeking to answer the research question: 'What support did you receive from the responding paramedic crew?' Clearly the REC will scrutinise this proposal most carefully. This study could be a useful contribution to knowledge and may lead to improvements in care delivery. However, the study would need to be conducted with great sensitivity as recounting the incident will lead to distress. The researcher must identify how this will be dealt with:

- Are there counselling services that the researcher could refer the parents to?

- What support is the researcher receiving to help them deal with the experience of hearing such sad narratives?

- How will the benefits of the findings from this study compare with the high potential for emotional distress?

Mental health considerations

The Mental Capacity Act 2005 protects those who lack mental capacity and offers protection for those unable to give informed consent by requiring that their previous wishes are respected and taking advice from those who know the person (DH 2005; IRAS 2009). Seeking to approach participants who are subject to the Mental Capacity Act requires particular sensitivity but mental illness is not an automatic barrier to research participation (Griffith and Tengnah 2010). To automatically exclude those with mental health issues from research participation can be yet another form of discrimination that this client group can experience.

Privacy and confidentiality

The rights of individuals to privacy and rights to confidentiality are important considerations during research studies. Privacy relates to our right to protect personal or private information from misuse or unauthorised disclosure. We take seriously our right to privacy and there are laws that help us maintain our privacy: 'a right to respect for privacy and family life' is Article 8 of the European Convention on Human Rights (Liberty 2008). We would not like a newspaper to investigate our personal lives and to use our intimate information to write an article without our permission. Neither would patients or their relatives!

Breach of confidence relates to a common law tort that protects private information that was given in confidence. If I used personal information conveyed to me by a patient as part of the paramedic–patient relationship I would have committed a breach in my duty of confidentiality to the patient if I shared it with others. As the HPC (2007: 5) notes the paramedic must:

- be able to practise within the legal and ethical boundaries of their professions

- understand the importance of and be able to maintain confidentiality.

Health records are examples of confidential information and paramedics have a contractual and professional responsibility to keep patients' information confidential, although such information will of course be shared within in the healthcare team appropriately (Harris and Cowland 2008).

Confidentiality is not, however, secrecy. If confronted with research data or other information that places research participants or others at serious risk of harm then the researcher has a legal and moral duty to breach confidentiality. This is a rare occurrence.

The Data Protection Act

Researchers must ensure that their actions do not contravene the 1998 Act when they are seeking to use potential participants' data. The Act requires that those who handle personal data do so in accordance with the Data Protection (Caldicott) Principles (Liberty 2009). In summary this Act requires that a person's data cannot be collected, stored, retrieved or organised without that person's consent. Additionally, data held for one reason cannot be then used for another unrelated purpose and data must not be kept for longer than is necessary for the purpose that caused its collection.

Researchers holding data must ensure that the confidentiality of this information is maintained, that data collected are only used for the purpose that the participant agreed to, and that data are destroyed as indicated in the research proposal (DH 2005). It must be made clear to participants just who will be accessing the data when providing information about the study prior to gaining consent. Systems must be in place so that personal information and data cannot be accessed, either intentionally or by accident, by those who have no right to do so. Raw data collected during a research study such as questionnaires or interview transcripts must be kept locked away or if data are held on computers they must then protected by secure password access.

Assuring anonymity

The researcher must ensure that there are measures in place that will assure participants' anonymity (Blaikie 2000). In many quantitative studies such as randomised double blind controlled trials, participants (usually called subjects in quantitative studies) are recorded by a coded number known only to the research leaders or to a statistical contributor. Published results are recorded in statistical overviews rather than by using individual responses and so the identity of the subject is relatively easily safeguarded. In qualitative studies, which use as data the actual words or behaviour of participants, ensuring anonymity for participants is more complex. Typescripts of interviews and any published data (qualitative research reports will use interview extracts to support the claims of the study) must be made anonymous by using pseudonyms and removing any information that would identify a person or a particular setting. A process of aggregation may be used whereby the data is reproduced with small changes made, such as removing identifying material that does not affect the message of the extract, so that individuals cannot be identified.

These legal requirements are pertinent to the conduct of research and the researcher must demonstrate that the research strategy does not contravene these demands. As has been noted earlier the paramedic tending a patient does not have the right to at the same time collect research data or specimens if the only consent gained was for treatment. Likewise, patients whose data were collected for one reason, such as a hospital admission, have a legal right to expect that the information is stored securely and not used for some other purpose such as research without their consent. The demarcation between research, clinical audit and service evaluation often seems blurred and although there can be ethical considerations for all, it is only research that requires REC approval (NREC 2007). Research is defined as 'the attempt to derive generalisable new knowledge including studies that aim to generate hypotheses as well as studies that aim test them' (NREC 2007: 2). Clinical audit and service evaluation does not include any intervention but rather measures merely what is already there. Patient data can then be drawn upon for such audit and service evaluations without consent, provided patient anonymity is preserved and access to this data is consistent with the requirements of the Data Protection Act.

Veracity and fidelity

Researchers are in a privileged position of access and this then requires of them particular responsibilities related to how they interact with and treat participants. Participants have a legal and ethical right to expect that they can trust the researcher to act in an honest manner with them and to treat them with respect. Veracity relates to the ethical requirement to be truthful when accessing participants and to maintain this principle when the study is in progress. Fidelity is a closely related ethical principle that requires that the researcher does not do anything that would compromise the relationship of trust that the participant has with the researcher.

If unprofessional or unlawful behaviour or practices are witnessed during a research study the researcher, especially if a health professional, has to make a decision about what to do with this knowledge. As the HPC (2008: 8) reminds us 'you must not do anything, or allow someone to do anything, that you have good reason to believe, will put the health or safety of a service user at risk'.

Clearly any behaviour witnessed that could cause harm or distress to patients or relations must be stopped and reported promptly to an appropriate body: this commitment would have been made clear to participants at the commencement of the study. The researcher has however to balance ethical and professional demands against wanting to remain in the field and maybe gaining insights that will improve care in the future.

Researchers are never above the legal and moral codes that society requires of all of its citizens but the ethical way to proceed in a research study is not always 100 per cent clear. Ethical codes are essential for the protection of research participants but they are not rules of conduct: they merely guide ethical research behaviour. The researcher who departs from an ethical research principle should only do so if they acknowledge the principle and fully justify any departure from the 'ought' of the principle (Denscombe 2002). The researcher is in a privileged position when individuals give of their time and trust to provide data for the study. The researcher must not consider participants as merely a means by which to gather data if doing so compromises the participant's rights.

Non-maleficence

Non-maleficence (*primum non nocere*) is an ethical obligation not to inflict harm intentionally (and is often discussed alongside the ethical principle of beneficence that is an obligation to help others). Non-maleficence is a core underpinning principle informing the 1949 Declaration of Helsinki (WMA 2008). Research studies must be designed so that risk of harm or injury to participants is avoided and if there is any such risk participants are aware of this potential. As has been noted earlier, risks to participants may involve psychological harm and measures must be in place to minimise this and to offer support. In clinical practice, as in research practice, just what we mean by 'harm' is not always totally clear. When I inject a patient with adrenaline he suffers harm (the needle punctures his skin and causes pain) but the overall consequences are good in that the patient does not go into anaphylactic shock. Likewise, ethical decisions during research are often not clear cut and require thoughtful and informed ethical deliberation (Griffiths 2008).

Conclusion

The rights of research participants to personal autonomy require that informed consent must be sought, the individual's right to privacy and dignity must be respected, harm must be avoided and researchers must be truthful and trustworthy in their dealings with research participants. If any of these principles are contravened then ethical research has not been undertaken. Attendance to the principles of research governance can help ensure that any research that paramedics are involved in is ethically appropriate. We have seen however that what is a correct ethical approach in a research study can be debated and may be situation specific. The study of ethical reasoning has a key place in the development of professional paramedic practice, especially when understanding the correct ethical approach to use when involved in or critiquing research.

References

Blaikie, N. (2000) *Designing Social Research*. Oxford: Polity Press.
Brewer, J.D. (2000) *Ethnography*. Buckingham: Open University Press.
Centers Disease Control and Protection (2009) *U.S. Public Health Service Syphilis Study at Tuskegee*. Available at: http://www.cdc.gov/tuskegee/timeline.htm [accessed 4 August 2009].
Cox, H., Albarran, J.W., Quinn, T. and Shears, K. (2006) Paramedics' perceptions of their role in providing pre-hospital thromobolytic treatment: qualitative study. *Accident and Emergency Nursing* 14(4): 237–244.

Denscombe, M. (2002) *Ground Rules for Good Research*. Buckingham: Open University Press.

Department of Health, Social Services and Public Safety (Northern Ireland) (2002) *Research Governance Framework for Health and Social Care*. Belfast: DHSSPS. Available at: www.dh.gov.uk [accessed 19 April 2010].

DH (Department of Health) (England) (2005) *Research Governance Framework for Health and Social Care* (2nd edn). Available at: www.dh.gov.uk [accessed 8 August 2009].

Goldkind S.F., Sahin, L. and Gallauresi, B. (2010) Enrolling pregnant women in research. Lessons from the H1N1 Influenza pandemic. *New England Journal of Medicine* 362: 2241–2243.

Gillon, R. (1986) *Philosophical Medical Ethics*. Chichester: Wiley.

Griffith, R and Tengnah, C. (2010) *Law and Professional Issues in Nursing* (2nd edn). Exeter: Learning Matters.

Griffiths, P. (2006) Being a research participant: the nurse's legal and ethical rights. *British Journal of Nursing* 15: 386–390.

Griffiths, P. (2008) Ethical conduct and the nurse ethnographer: consideration of an ethic of care. *Journal of Research in Nursing* 13(4): 350–361.

Griffiths, P. (2011) The nurses' role on a Medical Assessment Unit: an ethnography. *Journal of Clinical Nursing* 20: 247–254.

Harris, G. and Cowland, S. (2008) Ethics and law for the paramedic. In: Blaber, A. (ed.) *Foundations for Paramedic Practice: A Theoretical Perspective*. Maidenhead: McGraw-Hill/Open University Press.

HPC (Health Professions Council) (2007) *Standards of Proficiency – Paramedics*. London: HPA. Available at: www.hpc-uk.org [accessed 23 August 2009].

HPC (Health Professions Council) (2008) *Standards of Conduct, Performance and Ethics*. London: HPA. Available at: www.hpc-uk.org [accessed 23 August 2009].

IRAS (Integrated Research Application System) (2009). Available at: https://www.myresearchproject.org.uk [accessed 23 August 2009].

Johnson, M. (2007) Criticising research from an ethical point of view. In: Long, T. and Johnson, M. (eds) *Research Ethics in the Real World: Issues and Solutions for Health and Social Care*. London: Churchill Livingstone, pp. 85–102.

Liberty (2008) *The European Convention on Human Rights*. Available at: http://www.yourrights.org.uk/yourrights/the-rights-of-defendants/the-european-convention-on-human-rights.html [accessed 11 September 2010].

Liberty (2009) *Overview of Data Protection Principles*. Available at: http://www.yourrights.org.uk/yourrights/privacy/data-protection/overview-of-data-protection-principles.shtml [accessed 16 August 2009].

Long, T. (2007) What are the ethical issues in research? In: Long, T. and Johnson, M. (eds) *Research Ethics in the Real World: Issues and Solutions for Health and Social Care*. London: Churchill Livingstone, pp. 47–62.

Mason, J.K. and McCall Smith, R.A. (1994) *Law and Medical Ethics* (4th edn). London: Butterworth.

Mason, S., Knowles, E., Freeman, J. and Snooks, H. (2008) Safety of paramedics with extended skills. *Academic Emergency Medicine* 15: 607–612.

Medical Research Council (2009) *Ethics and Research Guidance*. Available at: http://www.mrc.ac.uk/Ourresearch/Ethicsresearchguidance/index.htm [accessed 25 October 2009].

National Institute of Health. *Directives for Human Experimentation: the Nuremberg Code*. Available at: http://ohsr.od.nih.gov/guidelines/nuremberg.html [accessed 8 August 2010].

National Research Ethics Consultation (NREC) E-Group (2007) *Differentiating Audit, Service Evaluation and Research*. Available at: www.nres.npsa.nhs.uk [accessed 25 July 2010].

Perkins, G.D., Woollard, M., Cooke, M. et al. (2010) Prehospital randomised assessment of a mechanical compression device in cardiac arrest (PaRAMeDIC) trial protocol. *Scandinavian Journal of Trauma, Resuscitation and Emergency Medicine* 18: 58.

PHRU (Public Health Resource Unit) (2007) *Critical Appraisal Skills Programme*. Available at: http://www.phru.nhs.uk/index.htm [accessed 18 April 2010].

Scottish Executive Health Department (2006) *Research Governance Framework of Health and Social Care*. Edinburgh: Scottish Executive Health Department. Available at: www.dh.gov.uk [accessed 19 April 2010].

UK Clinical Research Collaboration (UKCRC) (2009) Home page. Available at: http://www. ukcrc.org [accessed 1 November 2009].

Welsh Assembly Government (2002) *Research Governance Framework of Health and Social Care in Wales*. Cardiff: Welsh Assembly Government. Available at: www.dh.gov.uk [accessed 19 April 2010].

Winch, S., Henderson, A. and Shields, L. (2008) *Doing Clinical Healthcare Research: A Survival Guide*. London: Palgrave Macmillan.

World Medical Association (2008) *Declaration of Helsinki – Ethical Principles for Medical Research Involving Human Subjects*. Available at: http://www.wma.net/e/policy/b3.htm [accessed 4 August 2009].

Useful websites

College of Paramedics https://www.collegeofparamedics.co.uk/about_us/structure/research_ and_audit_committee/

Conducting a critical literature review in paramedic practice

Gail P. Mooney

Learning outcomes for the chapter

By the end of this chapter the reader should be able to:

1   Define and identify the characteristics of a literature review

2   Carry out a literature search

3   Understand the principles of critically analysing the literature

4   Structure and write a literature review

Keywords

critical analysis
literature reviews
literature searching
referencing

Introduction

A literature review is an important part of any research study regardless of the purpose or size of the study and its importance to the quality of the study should not be underestimated. A review of the literature is carried out an early stage in the research process to gain an understanding of what is already known about the subject. As a student this might be the only part of a research process that you carry out as reviewing the literature is not just required as part of a research study. For example, a literature review may form a student's dissertation or a module assignment or be used when developing practice. The paramedic is required to review the literature in order to ascertain what the current best practice is. Carrying out a review of the literature requires the reviewer to follow a procedure of various steps which will often be time-consuming. Many practitioners find the prospect of carrying out a review of the literature quite daunting, but if done well and on a topic that you have a general interest in it can be an exciting discovery of new knowledge. A significant element of reviewing literature is the reader's ability to critically review the research studies. This chapter will provide you with an overview of literature reviewing and show you how to go about conducting a literature review of your own.

What is a literature review?

A literature review is a planned process to review the published literature on a given subject. The review should include a selection of both published and unpublished literature, on a specified topic (Moule and Goodman 2009). The final product is a critical evaluation and summary of the literature obtained. It should provide you, and the reader, with a review of the current knowledge on a given subject or topic. It may identify 'gaps' in research. When we use the term 'gaps' we mean that there is no or limited research in an identified topic. For instance, investigating paramedics' attitudes and experiences of higher education we may find research in that topic but research that was carried out only using a particular method. For example, paramedics' attitudes and experiences of higher education may have been ascertained using a questionnaire collecting quantitative data but there may not be any studies identified that took a qualitative approach. Therefore, a 'gap' in the literature may be justification for carrying out a research study – often authors will use the term 'paucity' to describe this limited evidence.

For those unfamiliar with literature reviewing it is useful to read well-presented literature reviews to get a feel for what good literature reviews look like. Your university lecturer may have published a literature review or will be able to give you examples of other literature reviews.

The purpose of a literature review

There are a number of reasons why we carry out a review of the literature. As highlighted earlier we may review the literature for research purposes to set the proposed study in the context of what is already known on the subject. So the review may be part of the research process to guide us in the research we wish to undertake or it may be part of the research being undertaken when we draw on literature to help discuss research findings. You may review the literature to see what research methods have been used related to the research topic, for example to find out what patients' views are on response rate times. As professionals, our practice should be evidence based therefore we need to review the literature to inform our practice. We may carry out a literature review to gain more knowledge in an area of practice, or/and to answer our own questions that arise from practice, for example when to give a patient oxygen. For whatever purpose a literature review is carried out, the main reason is to gain more knowledge about an identified topic. The review should not be an argument for your own personal perspective of interest and it certainly should not be biased. For example, if you felt that relatives should not be present when treating a patient you would be wrong to only search and review this literature and excluded the papers that stated relatives should be present. Also, it should not be a reporting of the literature that is solely descriptive or a presentation of a list of references. The main purpose of the critical review is to compare and contrast research studies, identifying similarities and differences in the discovered literature related to the topic being explored.

Identifying a topic

The first stage in conducting a literature review is to identify the topic. For example, you may wish to find out the experiences of student paramedics in training and compare your experiences with other paramedic students. Now, this is quite broad as a topic so you would need to focus it down – is it the students' experiences of clinical placement or is it their experiences in college that you want to find out about? If you decide you wish to know about their experiences in clinical placement what is it you want to know?

- Do you want to know about all areas of clinical practice?

- Will you focus on how they feel?

- Will you investigate how they go about making decisions?

- Are you interested in the relationships with their practice placement educator?

It is important that you do focus your topic of interest otherwise you will end up with thousands of articles. Once you have decided on your topic you may find it useful to discuss your ideas with colleagues or your university lecturer: this will help you to focus and to ensure that you are being realistic in your aims before you start your searching of the literature. There is no good or bad topic or questions to ask but you must remember you cannot ascertain an answer if the topic is too broad.

Searching the literature

You will not be expected to find every article or publication on your identified topic for your literature review. You will however be expected to find the most up-to-date literature. You may find it useful to visit your university library to make yourself familiar with some of the journals available. There are a number of electronic databases that you will be able to search via your university or workplace if you have access to a library electronically. An Athens account may be needed to access some of these databases; your librarian will be able to help you out with this. Table 5.1 lists a number of databases that you may come across.

Using electronic databases is the foremost tool to use to search for literature. There are other methods that you must combine with using these databases as not all literature will be listed. Although hand searching is time-consuming, useful literature can be found if carefully planned. Policies, strategies, patient information

Table 5.1 Electronic databases

ASSIA social sciences package
BioMed Central scientific articles in all areas of medicine and biology
CINAHL Full-Text nursing and allied health journals
Cochrane Library evidence based medicine
Maternity and Infant Care Database (MIDIRS) maternity and infant
PsycInfo psychology and related disciplines, such as medicine, psychiatry, nursing, sociology, education, pharmacology, physiology, linguistics, anthropology, business and law
PubMed US National Library of Medicine includes citations from MEDLINE and other life science journals for biomedical articles
Web of Knowledge mainly research articles

---

leaflets, circulars, newsletters, unpublished literature etc. often will not be identified through these databases. This literature is known as the 'grey literature'.

A search strategy needs to be drawn up. This is a plan of how you are going to carry out the search. You need to identify words that you will use to search the literature. These are known as search terms. Think about your topic and what are the best terms to use. What alternative words and synonyms can you use? For example if you are interested in pain you may use terms such as analgesia, pain control, pain relief. Once you have found appropriate articles look at the keywords the authors have used (the keywords are usually located under the abstract). The keywords they have used may be different to those that you have used. You can then try using these as your search terms.

Once you have identified your search terms, limitations to the search need to be identified. We have all been in situations where we end up with thousands of articles. This is why we need to set limitations. A usual rule of thumb is to search for publications five years back, and then if you do not obtain sufficient literature you can search back another five years (Bell 2007). You must remember once you start searching for literature more than five years old the text is becoming dated. However, there may be articles or books that we call 'seminal work'. This seminal work is text that has influenced practice or thoughts and theories on practice and despite being 'old' or 'dated' it is essential to use. Some of the papers that you have obtained may have used the same reference(s). If they have it is likely to be seminal work and it needs to be included in your literature review.

To do an effective search you need to draw up an inclusion and exclusion criteria:

- Do you want to look at English language only?

- Do you want to look at UK published literature only?

- Do you want to look at literature that has been published in the past five years?

- Do you want to look at research only?

- Do you only want to look at quantitative research?

- Do you want to look at a certain age group?

- Do you want to look at a certain injury?

You may have to expand your search if you have been too limiting in your search and find very little literature. At this stage you may have to seek help and advice from your university librarian. Always keep a record of your search: the search terms you have used, the databases you have used and the number of hits that you have had with each search. You will need to keep track of the databases you have used and the results of what you have found. You may be required in an academic assignment or a paper you are writing to describe and explain your search strategy.

These days most of the papers found will display an abstract that will give you an idea if the paper is suitable to be included in your review. The author(s) should clearly summarise the paper highlighting key issues in the abstract. The majority of databases will take you to the electronic article (as long as your university subscribes to the journal) where you can view before printing out. If the article is not available at your library you may have to request through interlibrary loans; you will need to find out who will pay for this request (each article can be approximately £6–£9). Always check with the librarian how long the interlibrary loan will take as it can take a numbers of weeks. There is no set number of how many papers should be included in a literature review but you must include all the papers that you think are important. Some of the papers may need to be discussed in more detail than others.

Critiquing the literature

When you have identified the papers that you want to include in your literature review you will now have to critically review them. Although we evaluate and make decisions around us every day you may find when you first start critiquing literature it is not as easy as you think and will take some practice. When we critically appraise a research paper we are identifying the strengths and weaknesses in relation to the research process of that study (Hek and Moule 2006). Not all papers that are published are of 'sound' research therefore it is important that you critically evaluate them. Critically appraising the research is not only about looking for the negative points in the study. You have to draw on the strengths and weaknesses and make sense of the research, concluding what it means to your research and practice.

There are many developed frameworks available to help you with your critiquing. The Critical Appraisal Skills Programme (CASP) has designed a number of frameworks for both quantitative and qualitative research (CASP 1993). When critiquing the literature the research process is followed asking pertinent questions. Below are some general questions that can be asked when appraising published research papers.

Getting started

You need to allow yourself adequate time to critique the papers; never underestimate how long it will take you. It can take some hours to critique one paper depending on the length and complexity of the study. In order to get a 'feel' of the paper you need to read the paper straight through. The second time you read it you need to start the critical analysis.

The abstract/summary

This section should clearly summarise the paper giving you a clear overview of the study. So while reading the papers we ask the following questions:

- Does it summarise the whole study?
- Does it include a background to the topic, aim/and objectives, hypotheses (if relevant), methods, sample size, results and conclusions?
- Is the paper relevant to your research or practice?
- Who is the author(s)? Have they appropriate qualifications and background to conduct such a study?

Introduction/background/literature review

This is where the author(s) will give usually a brief background and review of the literature. They should identify any 'gaps' in the literature and a clear rationale for their study.

The questions to ask while looking at the paper include:

- What is the background to the study?
- Is the literature review easy to locate?
- Does the review discuss literature directly relevant to the aims of the research?
- Have the author(s) critically reviewed the literature?
- Have they compared and contrasted the papers?
- Are most of the references from the past five years?
- Are the 'gaps' in the literature identified?

Aims and objectives

The paper needs to clearly identify the aims and objectives of the study. You will need to be focussing on the aims and objectives throughout the critique of the paper.

The questions to ask while looking at the paper include:

- Is it clear what the author(s) were trying to find?
- Do you think the aim is important and significant?
- Do the research objectives and research questions support this aim?
- Are the *variables* of interest clearly explained and is it possible to distinguish independent and *dependent variables*? (quantitative research)

Methodology

The methodology concerns the design of the research – how was the study carried out?

The questions to ask while looking at the paper include:

- Is the design qualitative, quantitative or mixed methods?
- Is the study design an experiment, a quasi-experiment or a survey? (quantitative research)
- If experimental – was it a double-blind study?
- Can you identify the variables?
- If it is qualitative research is this phenomenology/grounded theory/ ethnography/generic qualitative?
- Is the design appropriate to answer the research questions?
- Could you offer suggestions so that the design could be improved?
- Was there a pilot study? Were any changes made to the design or data collection tool following this?

Sample

The researcher(s) will not be able to include the total population. In this section you are looking to see what the research population is, whether the subjects/participants were chosen equitably and whether the final sample represents the total population.

The questions to ask while looking at the paper include:

- What is the study population?
- How was the sample chosen?
- Has the sampling approach been discussed e.g. purposive, random etc.
- Is the sample relevant to the study?
- What is the sample size?
- Is the sample size adequate?
- Did the author(s) justify the sample size?
- Did any participants choose not to take part?
- Did any participants withdraw? Is it clearly described why?
- Are statistical power considerations discussed? (quantitative research)
- Are inclusion and exclusion criteria described?
- Can the results be reasonably generalised on the basis of this sample? (quantitative research)

Data collection

The author(s) should clearly describe the data collection tool(s) used with a clear explanation and rationale of why they were chosen.

The questions to ask while looking at the paper include:

- What tool was used to collect the data? Questionnaire/interviews/observations?

- How was the data collection tool designed?

- How was the data collected? if questionnaires, how were they distributed? If interviews who carried out the interviews and where did they take place? Why was this location chosen? Is it a neutral place to the interviewer and the participant? Does this have any influence on the data collected? Is it explained how and why the data was collected?

- Is validity and reliability discussed? (quantitative research) Is plausibility, credibility and relevance discussed? (qualitative research)

Ethics

In this section you are looking to see if ethical considerations have been addressed. Are the participants compromised in any way and can they be identified? If they can, what difference will it make?

The questions to ask while looking at the paper include:

- Has informed consent been considered?

- Were the participants given information sheets and consent forms? If not why not?

- How was the participant/subject approached/recruited and was this appropriate?

- Is anonymity and confidentiality discussed? How was this established and maintained?

- How was the research explained to the participants?

- Has potential harm or benefit to the participants been considered?

- Have the ethical issues been sufficiently considered?

- Have the author(s) sought and gained ethical approval from the appropriate committee or organisation?

(See Chapter 4 for more information regarding ethics.)

Data analysis/results/findings

In this section the author(s) should be describing how they analysed the data and the measures they used to do this analysis. The results/findings should be clearly presented. The author(s) do not need to discuss their findings in this section but in qualitative research findings and discussion may be presented together.

Quantitative studies

To find out more about the attributes of quantitative research studies see Chapters 8 and 9 in this book.

The questions to ask while looking at quantitative papers include:

- Is it clearly explained how the data are analysed – what statistical tests have been used?
- Have inferential statistics been used?
- What were the tests of significance that established whether the results could have occurred by chance?
- At what level was the significance level set?
- Are non-significant results clearly indicated?
- Have confidence levels been discussed?
- Are the tables and figures clearly described in the text?
- Are the characteristics of the sample described?
- Has validity and reliability been addressed?

Qualitative studies

To find out more about the attributes of quantitative research studies see Chapters 6 and 7 in this book. The questions to ask while looking at qualitative research include:

- How was the analysis carried out?
- Was the type of analysis appropriate for the qualitative approach undertaken?
- Do the author(s) describe clearly how the categories and themes were derived from the data?
- Do they identify who carried out the analysis?
- Were more than the researcher involved in the analysis?
- Have they included all the data in the analysis?
- Is rigour discussed? How was it established?
- Were participants able to check the results?
- What actions have the author(s) taken to test the credibility of the findings?
- Have the author(s) considered the potential for bias?
- Do they discuss *reflexivity* and their role in the study's conduct?

Discussion, conclusion and limitations

In this section the author(s) will discuss their findings and interpret what they mean. Finally, they will draw up conclusions and will make recommendations for further research or clinical practice. The researcher(s) should identify any limitations of the study and if they have any negative connotations to the findings.

Discussion

- Does the discussion relate to the findings?

- Are any new issues discussed in this section that do not appear in the findings? The author should be relating the discussion to the findings.

- Could the data be interpreted in other ways?

- Have all the research questions been answered?

- Does the discussion address the research aim and objectives?

- Does the discussion incorporate literature to develop and enhance the relevance of the findings?

Conclusion

- What conclusions do the author(s) make?

- Are the conclusions consistent with the findings?

- Would you suggest alternative conclusions?

- Are theoretical and practical implications of the results discussed adequately?

- Are the suggested recommendations feasible?

- Are recommendations for clinical practice, education or further research made?

Limitations

- Have you identified any limitations of the study?

- Have the author(s) identified any limitations?

- Do these limitations affect the research?

Overall judgement

At the end of the paper you need to make an overall judgement of the research. You need to consider if there are implications for your practice.

- Is the research reliable enough to influence your practice?

- Has the research added anything new to what is already known?

Managing your references

To help you organise your work you will need to keep a record of all the papers that you have reviewed. There are a number of ways that you can record the references either in hardcopy or electronically. Index cards are useful for storing your references – however, this method is a little outdated. There are electronic referencing software packages available such as Endnote. You may have access to this programme through your university library. You can also keep records of the references in a Word document. This can be quite unwieldy to manage, especially as your reference list grows.

If you are reviewing a number of papers you need to keep a record of your critique of the papers that you have reviewed. Several of the critical appraisal tools have space for you to document your critique. Using a form as such as in Table 5.2 can be useful to record a summary of the papers reviewed.

Table 5.2 Record of summary example

Full reference of paper	Methods	Sample	Data collection tool	Data analysis	Results/ findings
Chen AL (2008) Randomized trial of endotracheal tube versus laryngeal mask airway in simulated prehospital pediatric arrest. *Pediatrics.* 122(2) e294–297.	Randomised crossover study	52 emergency medical technicians	Scenarios using two different devices	For each participant, data with the two devices were compared by using the paired t test The rates of complications of ETTs with LMA was analysed using X^2 analysis	In simulated paediatric arrests, the use of laryngeal mask airway, compared with endotracheal tubes, led to more rapid establishment of effective ventilation and fewer complications when performed by prehospital providers

Whichever system you choose to use you must ensure that you have a record of the papers you have reviewed. Once have read the literature the next stage is to present it in a coherent fashion.

The layout of the literature review

Basically a literature review consists of an introduction, a main body and a conclusion. This sounds quite simple but the layout needs to be planned well. Drawing

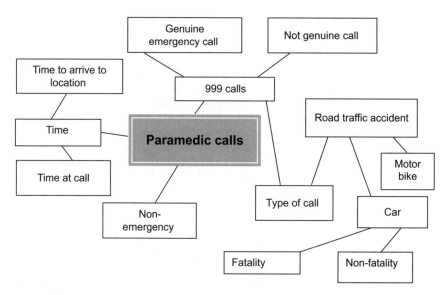

Figure 5.1 Example of a mind map

up a plan of your literature review will also help you to organise your writing. Mind mapping can be used to help you with the structure of the literature review and to map out the relationships between theories and concepts (Rowley and Slack 2004). A mind map is just a diagram of words that show relationships and links with one another. There is usually a central term. There is no right or wrong way to draw up a mind map. Having critiqued the papers you would have identified themes and trends in the literature. You are then documenting the themes that you have identified and looking at the relationship with one another. Throughout your review you will be comparing and contrasting the themes from the articles that you have reviewed. See Figure 5.1 for an example of a mind map. In this diagram you will see the central word is *paramedic calls*. The other words and terms are themes that emerged from reviewing the literature. The literature review should not be a list of the articles reviewed – reading as a 'shopping list' rather than as a carefully thought out and logical presentation of the literature.

The introduction

The introduction should include the aim of the review, the rationale and background. The introduction will be informing the reader of the content of the review. You will need to write a clear rationale explaining why you decided to undertake the review. The background should 'set the scene' for the reader, discussing relevant information. For example, what are the incidences of paramedic calls? Who coordinates the calls? Have there been problems with the calls that led you to this review? You may want to outline the structure of your review. The search strategy should be clearly described, identifying how you obtained your articles. It is often useful to highlight the number of hits the search obtained and how many articles you finally reviewed.

Reviewing the articles

The next stage is to write the review of the articles – demonstrating synthesis of the themes and concepts identified within them. Carnwell and Daly (2001) suggest the literature could be divided up into themes derived from the literature itself. Thus using the example from the mind map (Figure 5.1) the themes identified would be: paramedic calls, type of calls and duration of calls. The mind map identifies the concepts and the relationships between them. This conceptual framework will determine the organisation of your literature review. The review should draw out the key points and what you consider to be most important information from the literature. It may not be necessary to discuss and critique every paper in great depth, only the ones that have significance to your review. The key findings from the review need to be highlighted and discussed in your literature review.

Knopf (2006) suggests that the findings from a review can be divided into three categories: what the studies have in common; what they disagree about; and what they overlook. Throughout the review you will not only discuss the study's approach and findings but you will also point out its weaknesses and strengths. The critique of the studies is an essential part of reviewing the literature.

It is often viewed that a balanced argument needs to be presented in a review of the literature. If there are different views identified in the review of the studies then these do have to be presented in an impartial manner. The different views may not necessarily signal a disagreement but could have different findings as the researchers' approaches may have differed. You need to ask yourself if these views or findings are surprising to you and if so why. At this stage you need to critically discuss the differences and relationships between the concepts identified. Theories may become apparent as your review develops and these should be discussed in your review. The review should flow in a logical manner, linking each of the themes (concept) with one another.

Writing the conclusion

The conclusion draws the literature review to a close. A summary should be made of the review drawing on the main points and arguments made and providing an overview of current knowledge on a given subject. An emphasis of any 'gaps' in the literature may be re-emphasised here and these 'gaps' may include a lack of investigation into a topic using differing research approaches. Recommendations for further research may be discussed. The conclusion should provide a final statement of the core argument and represent approximately 10 per cent of the review (Redman 2006).

Referencing

You are required to identify your sources of ideas, data and other evidence in written work (Neville 2010). The reader of your work needs to identify what are your ideas and whose work you have used. Failure to do this is known as plagiarism. This can have serious consequences if you fail to credit other people's work and present it as your own. A reference list (which is always presented at the end of academic written work) is also useful for the reader of your work as it enables them to follow these references up. There are two main types of referencing styles: the Vancouver style and the Harvard style.

Vancouver style

The Vancouver system uses numbers in the text that then relate to the reference list, which is laid out in numerical order.

When citing an author in the text using the Vancouver style a number is used:

Additional studies are needed to establish LMA as a potential first-line device in the prehospital setting[1]

When citing using the Vancouver style the reference list is laid out numerically:

1 Chen AL (2008) Randomized trial of endotracheal tube versus laryngeal mask airway in simulated prehospital pediatric arrest. *Pediatrics*. 122(2) e294–7.

Harvard style

The Harvard style uses the author's name and date of publication in the text and the full reference is written alphabetically in the reference list.

When citing an author in the text using the Harvard style you use a name(s):

Chen (2008) states that additional studies are needed to establish LMA as a potential first-line device in the prehospital setting.

When citing using a Harvard style the reference list is laid out alphabetically:

Chen AL (2008) Randomized trial of endotracheal tube versus laryngeal mask airway in simulated prehospital pediatric arrest. *Pediatrics*. 122(2) e294–7.

You need to check which referencing style you need to follow before writing your literature review. Regardless of what style you decide to use it is important to keep an accurate record of all the references you have retrieved.

Conclusion

A literature review is generally a critical appraisal of existing knowledge on a given subject. It can be seen that reviewing literature has two main purposes: to inform clinical practice and to provide the foundations of a research study. There are a number of stages to go through in reviewing the literature: to define the aim or problem; develop a search strategy; critically review the literature; identify themes and concepts; and finally to write up the findings of the review. It is important to critically appraise the studies and not just systematically describe them.

Carrying out a literature review is an essential component of the research process. Researchers need to know what previous research has been conducted. The review will inform the researcher of the current position in a given subject. Also, the researcher will be able to identify any 'gaps' in the literature. Paramedics and other healthcare professionals need to deliver evidence based care so they need to rely on the literature to inform their practice. Ability in reviewing the literature in a critical manner plays a big part in helping inform paramedics how to best carry out their practice.

References

Bell, J. (2007) *Doing your Research Project* (4th edn). Buckingham: Open University Press.

Carnwell, R. and Daly, W. (2001) Strategies for the construction of a critical review of the literature. *Nurse Education in Practice* 1: 57–63.

Chen, A.L. (2008) Randomized trial of endotracheal tube versus laryngeal mask airway in simulated prehospital pediatric arrest. *Pediatrics* 122(2): e294–297.

Critical Appraisal Skills Programme (CASP) (1993). http://www.phru.nhs.uk/casp/casp.htm [accessed 29 January 2011].

Hek, G. and Moule, P. (2006) *Making Sense of Research: An Introduction for Health and Social Care Practitioners* (3rd edn). London: Sage.

Knopf, J.W. (2006) Doing a Literature Review. *Political Science and Politics* 39(1): 127–132. Available at: http://journals.cambridge.org [accessed 29 January 2011].

Moule, P. and Goodman, M. (2009) *Nursing Research: An Introduction*. London: Sage.

Neville, C. (2010) *The Complete Guide to Referencing and Avoiding Plagiarism* (2nd edn). Buckingham: Open University Press.

Redman, P. (2006) *Good Essay Writing* (3rd edn). London: Sage.

Rowley, J. and Slack, F. (2004) Conducting a literature review. *Management Research News* 27(6): 31–39.

Further reading

Aveyard, H. (2010) *Doing a Literature Review in Health and Social Care* (2nd edn). Maidenhead: Open University Press.

Hart, C (1998) *Doing a Literature Review – Releasing the Social Science Research Imagination*. London. Sage.

Hart, C. (2001) *Doing a Literature Search: A Comprehensive Guide for Social Sciences*. London: Sage.

Pears, R. and Shields, G. (2010) *Cite Them Right: The Essential Referencing Guide* (8th edn). London: Palgrave Macmillan.

Useful websites

http://www.sph.nhs.uk/what-we-do/public-health-workforce/resources/critical-appraisals-
skills-programme

http://medweb4.bham.ac.uk/websites/caspb/cribsheets/

http://www.sph.nhs.uk/what-we-do/public-health-workforce/resources/critical-appraisals-
skills-programme

6 Qualitative research in paramedic practice: an overview

Julia Williams

Learning outcomes for the chapter

By the end of this chapter the reader should be able to:

1 Understand the purpose of qualitative research

2 Outline core characteristics of qualitative research

3 Identify key stages in qualitative research

4 Discuss some of the challenges encountered when undertaking rigorous qualitative research in paramedic practice

5 Appreciate the role of qualitative research to inform and develop paramedic practice

Keywords

analysis
qualitative
reflexivity
research approach
trustworthiness

Introduction

The aim of this chapter is to introduce the potential for qualitative research in paramedic practice and to provide the reader with an overview to the key components of qualitative inquiry. Qualitative research facilitates our understanding of human experiences, and helps us learn more about human motivation, perceptions and behaviour. How individuals interpret experiences and attribute meaning to similar phenomena can vary between different people or, indeed, may change over time within the same person. Exploration of these similarities and differences requires flexibility in the approach to inquiry processes, and qualitative research design and methods afford opportunities to engage in systematic, robust exploration which is dynamic and adaptable.

What is the purpose of qualitative research?

When asked this question, people frequently indicate that it is a good way to find out about participants' attitudes, opinions and views and, on one level, this is the case. Qualitative research can establish this but examination of these areas can be achieved through quantitative questionnaires as well. Qualitative research has the potential to go so much further than merely reporting people's views and opinions. It encompasses a variety of ways to explore human behaviours, actions and experiences and provides opportunities to understand what people are doing and why. Qualitative research is not focussed on counting and measuring but, rather, it grapples with the essence of social phenomena and the meanings that individuals give to these events and processes. The qualitative researcher then offers an interpretation of their understanding in the research report.

A fundamental difference between qualitative and quantitative research is that qualitative research is inductive. This means that theory or interpretation emerges from the data rather than the researcher trying to *test* some external theory or prior interpretation from the outset. As the researcher's understanding develops through the processes of exploration and analysis of the data, so the emergent theory or interpretation takes shape.

Why choose a qualitative approach?

A qualitative approach should be chosen if it provides the most appropriate way to answer the research question. The focus of the research, the research problem, the research question(s) and aim(s) should drive the decision as to what is the most appropriate research design. Researchers should never pick their research methods first and then come up with a research question that *fits* the method.

If the researcher wants to *test* something or *prove causality* (something that causes another thing to happen) then a qualitative approach is not the way forward.

There are many reasons to use a qualitative research approach, for example:

- to increase understanding about topics about which little is known (also useful to further understanding about known topics)
- to explore people's perceptions, opinions, understanding and experiences of a variety of phenomena (see Box 6.1)
- to explore meanings that people give to their experiences
- to understand human motivation or behaviours
- to provide in-depth description about complex events and happenings
- to generate and/or develop theory.

Box 6.1 An example of a qualitative study in pre-hospital care

Forslund et al. (2008) explored the pre-hospital experiences of spouses of patients presenting with acute chest pain in order to understand what this emergency event is like for people on the receiving end of pre-hospital care.

This study was based in Sweden and interviews were used to collect data from 19 participants (13 wives and six husbands).

Very little is known about these events from the service-users' perspectives and having greater understanding about their experiences in these emergency situations may help paramedics in their development and delivery of targeted emergency care.

Characteristics of qualitative research

There is not just one singular approach to qualitative research; there are many different approaches (four of which are explored further in the next chapter). It is not surprising to find that there are some characteristics that may be unique to one specific qualitative tradition and not to others. However, Morse (1992) identifies three general characteristics of exploratory, qualitative research (a practical example of these is provided in Box 6.2):

• emic (insider) perspective

• holistic perspective

• inductive and interactive process of research inquiry.

Box 6.2 Practical application of Morse's characteristics of qualitative research

The research aimed to increase understanding of the relationship between the phenomenon of street homelessness and health (Williams 2006). The study focussed on the participants' understanding of health, illness and healthcare provision whilst living on the streets.

All three of Morse's characteristics are evident in the research:

• The study focussed on the participants' understanding and experiences (emic).

• Integral to the research aim was the exploration of the influence and impact of context (in this case sleeping rough on the streets) on the participants' lives (holistic).

• The research objectives emerged during the early days of fieldwork out on the streets with the growth of the researcher's knowledge and understanding of the participants' lives and immediate environmental contexts (inductive and interactive processes).

Morse describes an emic perspective as focussing on the participants' understanding and experiences rather than the researcher's theoretical beliefs and values: an inside perspective. Associated with this is a holistic perspective, which highlights the importance of the research context which influences individuals' experiences and construction of understanding. The third characteristic involving inductive and interactive processes of research inquiry emphasises the emergent and developmental nature of qualitative research.

Other characteristics associated with qualitative approaches, include:

- an exploratory approach and is often used when little is known about the subject

- a concern with understanding rather than prediction

- a cyclical, emergent and flexible design; as opposed to a linear and rigid one

- inductive processes in design and analysis

- data collection methods that are usually semi-structured or unstructured

- use of non-numerical data such as conversations from interviews/discussions, text, images etc.

- analysis that frequently includes elements of description and interpretation

- a focus on meanings that participants attribute to experiences

- a recognition that people may experience/interpret things differently; there is no one singular version of reality (concept of multiple realities)

- research undertaken in the participant's natural environment

- findings that are unique to the individual study but may have relevance to other settings (transferability)

- the researcher being active in all elements of the research processes and reflexivity is key.

Reflexivity

Qualitative researchers recognise that their presence and engagement in the research processes shape the study's development, and it is through their interaction and relationship with participants that the data are constructed. There is no one prescribed method to incorporate a reflexive approach within qualitative research and the issue is complex, but in essence:

> *reflexive research acknowledges that the researcher is part and parcel of the setting, context and culture they are trying to understand and analyst. That is to say, the researcher is the instrument of the research.* (Rice and Ezzy 1999:41)

A reflexive journal is a useful resource where researchers can note development of their ideas at all stages of the inquiry. It will contain all sorts of information including description of events, notations of a subjective nature, rationale for methodological decisions including those taken during processes of analysis.

Keeping a reflexive journal is an essential activity within qualitative research and its contribution to rigour is discussed later in this chapter.

What does a qualitative research study look like?

There is no one single configuration that neatly fits all qualitative research studies. However, although no two studies will be exactly the same, there are some shared characteristics. Qualitative research is seen to be more circular than linear in overall structure and process (Figure 6.1).

The rest of this chapter focusses on the different activities identified within this qualitative research cycle (Figure 6.1) using examples from existing paramedic literature to illustrate the points.

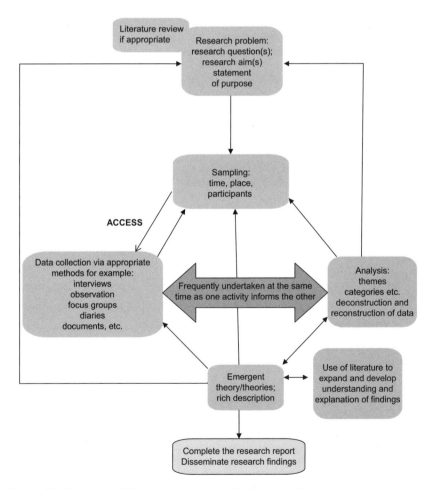

Figure 6.1 Illustration of dynamic activities in qualitative research

A cyclical model is used in qualitative research, rather than linear which you find used in quantitative studies (see Chapter 8), which provides opportunities for the researcher to revisit certain research activities (as indicated by the double-ended arrows in Figure 6.1) if more information and/or a different type of data are required to achieve the aim(s) of the study and answer the research question(s).

This does not mean that the qualitative researcher can lurch backwards and forwards randomly between the research activities, as there has to be a clear rationale for all of the research decisions. Qualitative research may be flexible but it has to be systematic and the process of decision making must be clearly documented by the researcher(s) to provide a transparent *audit trail* of the research.

Research problem, question and aim/statement of purpose

A clear statement of the research problem is needed to put the research in context. The explanation of the research problem usually draws upon existing literature and what is already known about the topic area and justification for undertaking the research. Depending on the research approach taken, there are differences as to when and how the research questions are developed. For example, the research questions may not be specified at the beginning of the study as they may emerge at later stages in the research process. Creswell (2009) suggests that the research question in qualitative research should be the broadest question that can be asked that is relevant to the study so as not to prematurely close off any potential avenues of inquiry.

Sometimes in published papers on qualitative research the research question is not explicitly stated with authors more frequently stating the aim or purpose of the study. Halter et al. (2011), who designed a clinical assessment tool (CAT) to help paramedics decide about conveyance to hospital for older adults who have fallen, identify both the question and aim for the qualitative components of their study (see Box 6.3). You will note that there are similarities between the research

---

Box 6.3 Examples of a qualitative research question and aim

Halter et al. (2011) clearly set the parameters of the research within their aim:

> to understand the decision making processes of emergency ambulance staff with older people who have fallen. (p. 44)

The research question is:

> What are the processes used by ambulance staff in the assessment of older people who have fallen? (pp. 44–45)

The qualitative aspects of the research were undertaken after ambulance staff had been using the CAT for six months. To answer this research question Halter et al. used semi-structured interviews with 12 ambulance staff (1 paramedic; 11 emergency medical technicians) to gather data enabling them to explore in depth the decision making processes employed by the participants when attending these calls.

question and the aim of the study, but the way they are written is different. The aim is written as a statement of intent; and the question is presented in an interrogative sentence. The two complement each other by giving the reader a more comprehensive picture of the overall purpose and focus of the study. The aim (or statement of purpose) should clearly identify the parameters of what is being researched and who is involved, and the central research question(s) should start to refine the focus of inquiry.

Sampling

Selecting people to participate in qualitative research can be done in a variety of ways. Qualitative research needs its participants to be able to make meaningful, knowledgeable contributions so it is likely that they will have experienced the phenomenon under exploration.

As can be seen from Evans et al.'s study (Box 6.4), purposive sampling involves the researcher recruiting from people who are known to meet the criteria of the study and who can talk from personal experience of the phenomenon under investigation.

Box 6.4 An example of purposive sampling within a qualitative study

Evans et al. (2010) explored the patient's handover by paramedics to the trauma team. They recruited 27 participants (10 paramedics; 17 trauma staff) all of whom had experience of these events:

> Purposive convenience sampling of paramedics and trauma team members was undertaken... Paramedics were sampled from the Mobile Intensive Care Ambulance (MICA) Air Wing and three paramedic stations in metropolitan Melbourne. All had some experience transporting critically injured trauma patients to a trauma service. Trauma team doctors and nurses were sampled to ensure representation from specialty groups involved in the immediate management of trauma patients in the Trauma Centre. (p. 2)

Purposive sampling is a form of non-probability sampling in that we do not seek to make statistical inferences. Other such approaches include:

- snowball sampling – where participants recommend someone else to participate (sometimes called nominated sampling)

- volunteer sampling – where people perhaps see an advertisement about the study and volunteer to participate

- convenience sampling – which can be seen in this study where the researchers recruited staff linked to the trauma centre who were easy to access.

Researchers and those conducting research critiquing need to be aware of the specific strengths and limitations of all of these individual strategies but overall they need to balance the principles of *appropriateness* and *adequacy* when making decisions about sampling (Morse and Field 1996). Appropriateness is guided by which participants can best contribute relevant data, and adequacy is achieved when the researcher has sufficient data to construct a complete description of the phenomenon under examination and when no new information emerges during data collection (saturation).

Data collection

No matter whether the study is qualitative, quantitative or mixed-method research, data collection is a central activity in the inquiry process. Creswell (2009) identifies four broad types of data collection in qualitative research:

- interviews
- observation
- documents – including public documents (policies, patients' records etc.) as well as private documents (letters, diaries, journals etc.)
- audio and visual material and other artefacts (photographs, music, videos, art, film, software etc.).

Most of the pre-hospital qualitative research to date has used different types of interview, and/or observation to collect data, and it is these more frequently used methods that will be expanded on in this overview chapter.

Interviews

Interviews provide an excellent opportunity to talk to the participants and to learn about their experiences, understanding and interpretation of the issues under investigation. Interviews in qualitative research are usually semi-structured or unstructured and are frequently audio recorded. Interviews may be undertaken:

- on a one-to-one basis either in person, over the phone, or via the internet
- in the form of a focus group.

Types of interview

1   Semi-structured, individual interviews enable the researcher to ask each participant the same core of questions but they also allow for researchers to follow up on areas that emerge during the interview to increase exploration around the research questions (Box 6.5).

Box 6.5 An example of a qualitative study using semi-structured interviews

In a small-scale qualitative study, Jones and Machen (2003) used semi-structured, individual interviews with six paramedics exploring their perceptions of patients in pain
and the factors which influence how they manage their patients' pain. By adopting this
approach, they asked the same nine questions to each participant but participants also
had the opportunity to raise new ideas as the interviews progressed.

2 Unstructured, individual interviews have no predetermined questions but
   rather the researcher starts with a broad open question as in the Forslund et al.
   (2008) study referred to earlier:

   *'Please tell me about the call you made to the EMD [Emergency Medical Dispatch]
   Centre.' (p. 234)*

   The researchers then followed up with other questions according to the participants' responses, such as:

   *"What did you do then?', 'Tell me more about that' and 'What was your experience
   of the contact you had with the ambulance personnel?' (p. 234)*

   Clearly these interviews can be intense events (both for the participant and
   the interviewer) and it is important that the researcher can devote their full
   attention to the participant, which is why it is common to audio record interviews as writing notes during an interview can be very distracting for both
   parties.
   Interviews are dynamic, complex interactions which have the potential to
   uncover rich data, but they are not without their challenges (see Table 6.1).

Table 6.1 Examples of the strengths and limitations of individual interviews

Strengths	Limitations
Protected individual time for the participant so that they can talk without being influenced by others	Time-consuming to carry out
If mechanically recorded, there is consistency in the documentation of data	Time-consuming to prepare for analysis if they are recorded, as the audio files need to be transcribed into a written record
If participants do not understand the questions, the researcher can rephrase them	Not all participants can put their feelings and experiences into words succinctly
The researcher has the opportunity to explore issues raised in the interview with each individual	Unstructured interviews can be challenging to analyse as participants are not asked the same questions and each interview can produce very different information

3 Focus groups (sometimes referred to as interviews for example, Creswell 2009) are group discussions usually involving somewhere between four and twelve participants. More than this is considered too many as people may struggle to get their ideas across in the allocated time, and less than this may make it difficult to sustain the conversation depending on the individual participants. Some of the benefits of focus groups include:

- participants can share experiences and 'bounce' ideas off each other
- opportunity to gain a variety of different participants' perspectives within one event
- ability to gather breadth of information within one event
- dynamic event which can help participants recall things they may not have thought of in an individual interview.

Some of the challenges that can be encountered with focus groups:

- getting several participants in one place at one time – particularly challenging if you have to get frontline ambulance staff stood down from shift to participate
- sometimes there can be individuals who dominate the discussion so a skilled facilitator is required to oversee the focus group to make sure everyone has an opportunity to contribute
- information gained may be superficial
- confidentiality may be at risk especially as the researcher cannot control what participants say to other people once they have left the focus group venue.

Despite these challenges focus groups as a research method in pre-hospital emergency care settings is popular (Box 6.6).

Box 6.6 An example of a qualitative research study using focus groups

Porter et al. (2008) undertook three focus groups with a total of 25 paramedics (6–10 in each group) to explore their experiences of and views about completion of clinical documentation, particularly relating to patients who were not conveyed. To avoid having to stand paramedics down from a shift, the researchers undertook the focus groups when paramedics were attending in-service training days.

Observation

Observation as a research method can be used on its own or as a supplementary method to complement information gained through other data collection methods such as interviews. Data collection often includes intensive documentation of field-notes recorded during periods of observation (see Box 6.7).

There are varying levels of participation (see Chapter 9) that the researcher can undertake when using observation as a research method, ranging from complete participant through to complete observer (Hammersley and Atkinson 1998).

Box 6.7 An example of a qualitative study using observation

Nurok and Henckes (2009) observed different approaches to pre-hospital care in New York ('scoop and run') and Paris, where clinicians were more likely to attempt to stabilise the patient on scene ('stay and play'). Through systematic analysis of the data (observation field-notes) it emerged that perceptions of pre-hospital emergency care work are shaped by the value that practitioners ascribe to the various activities that they undertake or the type of calls that they attend within their professional roles.

However, in many studies it seems that the researcher takes on a role that sits somewhere between the two extremes of this continuum.

Observation is a complex and time-intensive method of data collection and consideration must be given to various aspects including:

- gaining access to the research setting

- being accepted by the group – the 'insider/outsider' experience

- effective documentation of field-notes when in the 'field' for prolonged periods

- being aware that the researcher's presence might actually change the participants' usual behaviour

- getting too involved in the research setting and participants' culture so the researcher runs the risk of losing the focus of the study and 'going native'

- managing observation fatigue as the periods of observation can often be extremely intense for participants and researcher alike

- issues related to withdrawal from the research setting after prolonged periods of observation.

Approaches to analysis in qualitative research

Approaches to analysis in qualitative research are as varied as the overall research approaches themselves and should be guided by relevant traditions such as ethnography, phenomenology, grounded theory (discussed in Chapter 7). In this section, what is presented is an outline of some key principles of analysis in qualitative research. Specific frameworks, details and application of analytical techniques will be found in the many specialist texts written about approaches to qualitative data analysis.

What do we mean by qualitative data analysis?

Analysis is about making sense of the information (data) that has been collected. Rigorous processes of data analysis (see Box 6.8) involve taking the (potentially

Box 6.8 Overview of processes involved in qualitative data analysis

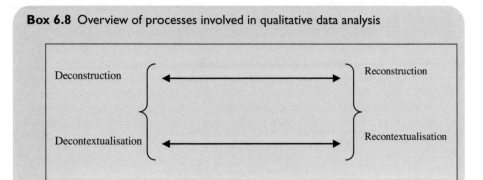

large) body of information (raw data) from all of the individual sources of data and:

• preparing the data so that they are in a usable, practical format for analysis

• breaking the data down into smaller, analytical units (deconstructing) which temporarily disassociates this data from the whole context of the research (de-contextualising)

• rebuilding (reconstructing) the data into larger meaningful units (categories; themes etc.)

• shaping the data (recontextualising) into something meaningful for the audience without compromising the truth of the participants' contributions.

This requires the researcher to be willing to immerse themselves in the data and to become totally familiar with the content of the data before starting active processes of analysis. These activities are very labour intensive and can be time consuming.

Whether or not to use software packages (often abbreviated to CAQDAS – Computer Assisted Qualitative Data Analysis Software) to assist in the analysis of qualitative data is often debated by researchers. Their use does not reduce the researcher's role in rigorous analytical development within qualitative data analysis as none of them do the analysis for you!

However, CAQDAS can help you to manage the data making it easier to:

• store data

• code data

• search data

• retrieve data.

In addition, CAQDAS is beneficial as it provides a transparent audit trail of the developments in analysis as the work progresses (see Table 6.1).

In qualitative research, data collection and data analysis are activities that frequently occur simultaneously; with one activity informing the other (this is called an iterative process). Before interpretive processes of analysis can begin, the data need to be prepared. For example, if data were obtained via recorded interviews then these recordings need to be transcribed (put into a written form) so the researcher has a tangible product to work with.

In general, qualitative data analysis is involved with exploring the data looking for patterns and similarities but just as important as the identification of emergent similarities is the recognition of differences that appear within the data sets. Exploring *atypical cases* (Morse and Field 1996) can be particularly enlightening and may provide opportunities for focussed exploration of areas relevant to the research that may otherwise have been overlooked.

Analysis is a creative process within qualitative research which may share some common features across the different qualitative approaches, but, also, it may be guided by method specific attributes as well. Researchers are required to keep detailed records of their decision trails throughout these activities and to make them available to others who may need to access this information when assessing the quality of the research study.

What is important in assessing the quality of research using qualitative approaches?

The constantly emerging literature relating to consideration of rigour within qualitative research continues to demonstrate a lack of consensus. Rolfe (2006) suggests that the debate divides broadly into three camps:

- use the same criteria to judge qualitative research as is used for quantitative research

- use different criteria to evaluate qualitative research

- discard the notion of generic criteria to assess all qualitative studies.

Lincoln and Guba's (1985) classic work on methodological rigour has influenced many writers in the realms of qualitative inquiry. Their concept of trustworthiness, which relates to the truth value of a study, can be established by using techniques to demonstrate *credibility, transferability, dependability* and *confirmability* (Erlandson et al. 1993):

- *Credibility* enhances trustworthiness through the acknowledgement of existence of multiple realities. The researcher has a duty to report the participants' perspectives as clearly, accurately and fairly as possible. Participants should be able to recognise and affirm any descriptions that the researcher constructs when presenting the findings of an inquiry (Lincoln and Guba 1985). Techniques to establish credibility include: prolonged engagement, triangulation, peer-debriefing, member checks and the use of a reflexive journal (see Table 6.2).

Table 6.2 Techniques to demonstrate elements of trustworthiness

Technique	Explanation and activities
Prolonged engagement	To increase credibility the researcher spends extended periods of time in the research setting to explore the context of the research, to learn about the participants, and to minimise the effect of any distortions that may have been caused by the presence of the researcher. Prolonged engagement helps in building trust relations between the researcher and the participant
Triangulation	Includes using different sources of data and/or different data collection methods to look at the same phenomenon but from different perspectives to increase the credibility of the data. Can also include using multiple researchers at various points in the study perhaps for data collection and/or analysis
Peer-debriefing	This covers a range of activities to increase credibility, including presenting at conferences and getting feedback about the research process and findings, getting peers to debate methodological issues, and involving peers in analytical procedures such as coding
Reflexive journal	Supports all aspects of trustworthiness in a study and can become an integral part of the audit trail
Member checking	Enhances credibility through getting feedback from participants. This could involve asking participants whether an interview summary is accurate and whether they want to add anything else before the interview finishes; or participants can be given copies of various parts of the research report to comment on the researcher's interpretation of the data; or perhaps the researcher might get a panel of participants to look at the entire report and give feedback to the researcher before releasing the report into the public domain
Thick description	Transferability can be enhanced by the provision of very detailed information about the environment and the participants. This level of detail frequently comes from field-notes from observation undertaken during the research. The detail should increase the readers' familiarity with the research so they can make sense of the findings and evaluate their potential for transferability
Purposive sampling	Involves the selection of participants who are believed to be able to give rich, robust information about the phenomenon being researched. They usually have had firsthand experience of the situation which increases the potential for transferability of the findings
Audit trail/Decision trail	Enables an external auditor to assess the dependability and confirmability of the research. It should include a record of all activities undertaken during the research. This may not be just written accounts such as field-notes, documents etc., but may include audio-visual recordings, photographs etc. If researchers have used CAQDAS the summary sheets from these software programmes are time/date stamped and make an effective contribution to the audit/decision trail

- *Transferability* relates to whether or not the findings are relevant to other settings or to other groups of people. The researcher needs to provide sufficiently detailed information about the participants and their contexts so that the reader can judge how transferable the findings are to other settings. Techniques for confirming transferability include: thick description, purposive sampling and the reflexive journal (see Table 6.2).

- *Dependability* pertains to whether or not the findings would be consistent if the study were carried out again with similar participants or in a similar setting. Of course, given an acceptance of multiple realities in qualitative inquiry there is likely to be some variance. Techniques for establishing dependability include: provision of a clear audit trail, and the reflexive journal (see Table 6.2).

- *Confirmability* is concerned with evidencing that the origins of the research findings can be tracked back to the original data. Researchers need to demonstrate clearly what has influenced their interpretation of the data, identifying potential and actual bias where it is known. Techniques for establishing confirmability include: the provision of an audit trail, and the reflexive journal (see Table 6.2).

Although the pursuit of rigour is important within qualitative research, it should not become a means to an end. There is no hard and fast rule as to how many of the activities listed in Table 6.1 are needed in a qualitative study. Researchers need to utilise appropriate techniques according to the study's needs. We would recommend that keeping a reflexive journal in qualitative research is important and that all qualitative researchers must be able to evidence a robust audit trail of their research.

Overall, it is a matter of establishing an acceptable balance between all the activities as, otherwise, there may be a danger of finding out more about the researchers (in the name of reflexivity) or the measures taken to promote rigour rather than learning about the actual research itself and the emergent findings of the study (Sandelowski and Barroso 2002).

Dissemination of the research findings

Once the research is completed, it is imperative that the findings are shared with other people (disseminated). It could be considered as unethical to carry out research without disseminating the findings. You should consider:

- Who needs to know about the research? For example,
  - healthcare practitioners
  - policy makers
  - health service providers
  - general public.

- How are they going to be informed? For example,
  - written papers
  - presentations at conferences, meetings, seminars etc.

These issues are discussed in more detail in Chapter 10.

Conclusion

The scope of qualitative research is immense and the different approaches within qualitative research are numerous. What is important is that researchers select the appropriate research approach and methods to meet the study's aim(s) and answer the research question(s). One of the risks of a broad chapter such as this one, which provides an overview of topic areas, is the danger of oversimplification of the issues. This chapter must be considered as a starting point, a springboard for further investigation before actually commencing a qualitative research study. As with any rigorous research, whether it is qualitative or quantitative, there are choices to be made with regards to methodological approach and methods, and these should be informed decisions taken from a position of knowledge and understanding.

This chapter has examined the role of qualitative research approaches and identified some of their common shared characteristics. The flexibility of this research approach has been illustrated and linked to research examples from paramedic practice as well as my own work on street homelessness. Not all qualitative research is the same and in the following chapter, four different qualitative research approaches are explored in more depth and linked to research in paramedic practice.

References

Creswell, J.W. (2009) *Research Design: Qualitative, Quantitative, and Mixed Method Approaches* (3rd edn). Thousand Oaks, CA: Sage Publications.

Erlandson, D.A., Harris, E.L., Skipper, B.L. and Allen, S.D. (1993) *Doing Naturalistic Inquiry: A Guide to Methods*. Newbury Park: Sage Publications.

Evans, S.M., Murray, A., Patrick, I., Fitzgerald, M., Smith, S. and Cameron, P. (2010) Clinical handover in the trauma setting: a qualitative study of paramedics and trauma team members. *Quality Safety Health Care* 19: 1–6 doi:10.1136/qshc.2009.039073.

Forslund, K., Quell, R. and Sørlie, V. (2008) Acute chest pain emergencies – spouses' prehospital experiences. *International Emergency Nursing* 16(4): 233–240.

Halter, M., Vernon, S., Snooks, H. et al. (2011) Complexity of the decision-making process of ambulance staff for assessment and referral of older people who have fallen: a qualitative study. *Emergency Medical Journal* 28(1): 44–50.

Hammersley, M and Atkinson, P. (1998) *Ethnography: Principles in Practice* (2nd edn). London: Routledge.

Jones, G.E. and Machen, I. (2003) Pre-hospital pain management: the paramedics' perspective. *Accident and Emergency Nursing* 11(3): 166–172.

Lincoln, Y.S. and Guba, E.G. (1985) *Naturalistic Inquiry*. Beverly Hills, CA: Sage Publications.

Morse, J.M. (1992) The characteristics of qualitative research. In: J.M. Morse (ed.) *Qualitative Health Research*. Newbury Park, CA: Sage Publications.

Morse, J.M. and Field, P.A. (1996) *Nursing Research: The Application of Qualitative Approaches* (2nd edn). Cheltenham: Stanley Thornes (Publishers) Ltd.

Nurok, M. and Henckes, N. (2009) Between professional values and the social valuation of patients: the fluctuating economy of pre-hospital emergency work. *Social Science Medicine* 68(3): 504–510.

Porter, A., Snooks, H., Youren, A. et al. (2008) Covering our backs: ambulance crews' attitudes towards clinical documentation when emergency (999) patients are not conveyed to hospital. *Emergency Medical Journal* 25(5): 292–295.

Rice, P.L. and Ezzy, D. (1999) *Qualitative Research Methods: A Health Focus*. Melbourne: Oxford University Press.

Rolfe, G. (2006) Validity, trustworthiness and rigour: quality and the idea of qualitative research. *Journal of Advanced Nursing* 53(3): 304–310.

Sandelowski, M. and Barroso, J. (2002) Finding the findings in qualitative studies. *Journal of Nursing Scholarship* 34(3): 213–219.

Williams, J. (2006) Street Homelessness: People's Experiences of Health and Healthcare Provision. Unpublished doctoral dissertation, University of London.

7 Using qualitative research methods in paramedic practice

Julia Williams

Learning outcomes for the chapter

By the end of this chapter the reader should be able to:

1   Identify the key characteristics of four different approaches in qualitative research

2   Recognise methodological challenges within these different approaches

3   Outline examples of qualitative research linked to paramedic practice within each of these approaches

4   Describe the potential for research in paramedic practice for each of these different approaches

Keywords

ethnography
generic qualitative research
grounded theory methodology
phenomenology

Introduction

From the previous chapter it is clear that there is not just one approach within qualitative research. Making a decision about what is the most appropriate way forward to answer a qualitative research question requires the researcher to know about the different approaches within qualitative inquiry. Before embarking on a qualitative study for the first time the researcher should find time to talk to people who have undertaken qualitative research to see what challenges confronted them and how they navigated their way through the research. Sharing experiences is a great way to learn about practical aspects of research and it helps to shape our understanding of research approaches. If you are reading this chapter to help you critique or understand research papers then ask all the time: is this a suitable approach to answer the research question?

This chapter provides an outline of four common approaches in qualitative research that have been used in pre-hospital research:

- ethnography

- grounded theory

- phenomenology

- generic qualitative research.

It is beyond the scope of this text to equip a researcher with a sufficient knowledge to undertake a study using any one of these approaches but this chapter will introduce the overall characteristics of each approach. If you are critiquing a research article that states that a certain qualitative approach has been used then look for the core characteristics of the approach in the research paper.

How do you choose the 'right' research approach?

Sometimes there is considerable pressure on qualitative researchers to give their research a label such as ethnography, grounded theory or phenomenology even if it does not completely fit the study's aim(s). As discussed in Chapter 6 the researcher needs to select an approach which provides the best chance of answering the research question(s) and addressing the area under investigation. The most important factor in the final decision should be whether or not the philosophy underpinning the selected research approach is appropriate and meaningful to the study.

To be able to make a choice, the researcher needs to know what the options are and what they actually mean. Throughout the rest of this chapter we will take each of these four research approaches (ethnography, phenomenology, grounded theory, and generic qualitative research) and identify the associated tradition which has informed the development of the approach. Then using real examples of research studies we will demonstrate the key features of the individual research approaches by:

- highlighting the focus and purpose of the research approach

- identifying common methods of data collection used within the research approach

- illustrating key concepts attributed to the research approach

- discussing some practical considerations relevant to the approach.

Ethnography

A central tenet of ethnography is the phenomenon of culture. Ethnography is an approach that has developed from anthropology (Box 7.1) where researchers

Box 7.1 Characteristics of ethnography

Tradition anthropology
Focus study of culture and influences of culture on behaviour
Common methods of data collection intensive observation (varying degrees of participation); interviews; study of documents and/or artefacts
Key concepts thick description; reflexivity; immersion in culture; prolonged engagement; becoming an 'insider'; fieldwork; telling the story
Practical considerations insider/outsider relationship; overt vs. covert research; challenges of prolonged engagement including 'going native'; researcher as self

N.B. You may not find all of these characteristics in every ethnography

would literally live within the society or with the group that they were studying to learn about all aspects of the group's culture in order to understand how people's behaviour is shaped and determined by the culture in which they live.

The main data collection methods within ethnography are participant observation and interviews involving extensive fieldwork and prolonged engagement. Other data sources such as documents, diaries, electronic communications and photographs can all provide useful contextual data within ethnography. Lincoln and Guba (1985) argue that periods of prolonged engagement are important in establishing the credibility of a study and this technique is particularly relevant to ethnography.

Prolonged engagement occurs when a researcher spends time with the research participants in their own environments and social contexts. Not only does this help to construct a rapport between researcher and research participants, but eventually it balances out any unusual occurrences or reactions that may occur in response to the researcher's presence, particularly in the early days of the research. The idea is that, when participants get used to the researcher being around, if participants' behaviour had changed when the researcher was new to the environment, over prolonged periods of time they will revert to their 'normal' behaviour. It is important that ethnography occurs in the participants' natural setting rather than creating an artificial environment to carry out the research. This is clearly demonstrated in the following example.

An example of ethnography in paramedic practice

An ethnography focussing on paramedics and emergency medical technicians (EMT) was undertaken in the United States to explore the cultural influences on occupational behaviour (Palmer 1983). Although, Palmer's research was published 28 years ago, it is notable how certain aspects of the study still demonstrate transferability today, for example, what type of emergency call is valued, and what is seen as an inappropriate use of emergency ambulance services.

It is evident that this research engaged with a variety of data collection methods aligned with ethnography and Palmer identifies which ethnographers informed the development of his research:

> *Data were gathered by participant observation, direct observation, informal interviews, conversations, listening to official radio traffic, and inspection of written documents obtained through immersion into the work culture . . . Thus data are basically qualitative in nature (obtained overtly) and were gathered in the ethnographic traditions espoused by Lofland (1976) and Manning and Van Maanen (1978).* (Palmer 1983: 164)

So Palmer used classic methods associated with ethnography through prolonged periods of fieldwork including observation, informal interviews and conversations. He supplemented this with other data collection methods including exploration of documentation. Through spending over 500 hours in the setting he became immersed in the culture and even qualified as an EMT. He uses the field-notes of his observation as a primary source of data and includes extracts of his notes in his published paper. Palmer engaged in different levels of participant observation during the study, at times even providing emergency care to patients as he became accepted as part of the team. He appears to cross over from 'outsider' status to 'insider' status as the participants become used to him being around.

There are several interesting features about Palmer's paper. For example, the style in which it is written is very much a narrative description, almost like a story rather than a structured research paper of today where the standard presentation includes:

- introduction

- literature review

- methods

- analysis

- results/findings

- discussion

- conclusion.

Hammersley and Atkinson (1983) emphasise that there is no one way to write an ethnography and that ethnographers need to find a style that enables them to narrate their findings in a way that most accurately reflects the participants' realities. Creswell (2007) argues that this open style may be disconcerting to people used to a more traditional structure to reporting research studies. However, in his writings, Palmer achieves detailed, thick description which contributes to enhanced rigour through transferability (discussed in Chapter 6) as it enables the reader to judge for themselves whether the researcher's interpretation is plausible.

Another interesting disclosure is that his research was overt as opposed to covert. Simply this means that Palmer did not try to hide his research activities from his participants. Covert research is when the research is done almost 'undercover' which involves an element of deception on the researcher's part. There are clearly ethical issues involved in covert research and where possible it is discouraged (see Chapter 4). If Palmer wanted to undertake covert research presumably he would have trained as an EMT before starting the research and then worked as an EMT while discreetly gathering data without his colleagues knowing that he was engaged in research.

Palmer's research (Box 7.2) culminates in the production of an insightful narrative about everyday life on the road for paramedics and EMTs in an urban ambulance service in the United States.

Box 7.2 Evidence of characteristics relevant to ethnography in Palmer's study

Focus: Palmer explores cultural influences on occupational behaviour of paramedics and EMTs within an ambulance service. The study is carried out on-the-road in a pre-hospital setting, which for this study is an appropriate natural setting.

Methods of data collection: Palmer combines observation (different levels of participant observation); interviews; examination of written documents; and listening to radio calls to collect data. He does not rely just on one source of data. All of these methods fit with ethnography, providing rich data for analysis.

Key concepts: Palmer immersed himself in the culture by actually working as an EMT which was a good way to maintain prolonged engagement in the field. He worked as part of the team and it appears he became accepted as an 'insider'. Palmer adopts a narrative style in the writing of the report, which makes the reader feel like they are in the research setting. He provides detailed information known as 'thick' description so that we can visualise what was happening out on the road. This narrative helps us to evaluate how relevant his findings are, if at all, to our own settings.

Practical considerations: Palmer chose to undertake overt research which meant that his work colleagues knew he was doing the research. Undertaking ethnographic research is time intensive. Palmer spent over 500 hours familiarising himself with the setting as well as collecting data. When planning a study you need to consider the financial costs of the various types of research and how it will be funded.

Verdict on Palmer's research – ethnography or not?

YES

Phenomenology

Phenomenology aims to achieve a rich understanding of individuals' life experiences and it is concerned with staying true to these experiences (Creswell 2007). Phenomenology emphasises the importance of seeing things from the participants' perspectives and to understand how they feel. It is a popular approach within healthcare research but is not without its challenges partly due to the different types of phenomenology and researchers' varied interpretations of processes within phenomenology.

Box 7.3 Characteristics of phenomenology

Tradition philosophy
Focus understanding human experience and its attributed meaning
Common methods of data collection usually unstructured interviews; could include diaries; letters; photographs
Key concepts lived experience; detailed description; bracketing; participants must have experienced the phenomenon under exploration; multiple realities
Practical considerations can be lengthy interviews often unstructured; challenges to suspending researcher's own experiences in order to most accurately describe the participants' views and experiences; different schools of phenomenological thought

N.B. You will not find all of these characteristics in every phenomenology

Historically this approach emerged from philosophy (Box 7.3). Flood (2010) indicates the core focus of phenomenology is to understand human experience as expressed by the individuals themselves.

There are two major approaches within phenomenology:

- *Descriptive:* associated with one of the early phenomenologists, Edmund Husserl (1859–1938), who believed the essence of the lived experience could be accessed through human consciousness

- *Interpretative:* often referred to as hermeneutic phenomenology, which goes beyond the descriptive and seeks to look for meanings that individuals attribute to their lived experiences (Heidegger 1962).

A particular difference between these two strands of phenomenology is engagement with a practice known as *bracketing*, which came from Husserlian phenomenology:

Simply described, it means the 'suspension' of the researcher's preconceptions, prejudices and beliefs so that they do not interfere with or influence [his/]her description of the respondent's experience. (Parahoo 2006: 68)

So bracketing literally means to put brackets round the researcher's experiences, and to suspend them so that their experiences and views do not influence how they report the participants' experiences. There are many challenges to being able to do this as it is hard to set our own feelings/opinions/experiences to one side. However, within descriptive phenomenology, bracketing is encouraged to help the researcher to describe the participants' experiences as accurately as possible.

On the other hand, hermeneutic phenomenology actively discourages bracketing, recognising that both researcher and participant have their own life experiences and preconceptions. It may not be possible (or desirable) to completely block these out but it is important to be aware of them and the impact they may have on our interpretation of events.

An example of a phenomenological study in paramedic practice

Elmqvist et al. wanted to understand more about patients' experiences of the first time they came into contact with pre-hospital emergency care services. The aim of the research was 'to describe and understand the patient's first encounter with pre-hospital emergency care as experienced by the patient and the first responders' (2008: 186).

In total, 18 people participated in unstructured interviews which allowed the researchers to gather in-depth information about participants' experiences of their first pre-hospital encounter relating to traumatic injuries. Participants included:

- 4 patients
- 3 ambulance staff
- 2 firemen
- 8 policemen
- 1 next of kin.

The research was carried out in Sweden where different emergency services are more frequently involved in the first response to medical emergencies than in the UK. Not all research findings are appropriate to every country/culture so readers need to look for the potential for transferability within the research findings and decide which, if any, elements are useful to them.

Within their analysis, Elmqvist et al. aimed to uncover meanings of the participants' lived experiences of this phenomenon. They acknowledge their attempts at bracketing their own experiences (they refer to it as a need to *bridle* their own preconceptions) in order to accurately represent the participants' accounts. They clearly detail the procedural stages in their analysis making reference to known writers in the field of phenomenology who influenced their approach such as Giorgi (1997).

The findings describe the essence of the experience of the patients' first encounter, which was often reported as chaotic. Five constituent elements emerged which emphasise the variations in participants' experiences: 'the encounter with the helpless injured body, the confirming existential encounter, the encounter while waiting, the lived encounter and the recapitulated encounter' (2008: 185).

From the data generated by using this research approach (Box 7.4), Elmqvist et al. concluded that being a patient in an emergency situation can be a disempowering and distressing experience. Emergency care providers need to find ways to provide emotional support to these patients whilst at the same time delivering appropriate urgent medical treatment.

Box 7.4 Evidence of characteristics relevant to phenomenology in Elmqvist et al.'s study

Focus: Elmqvist et al. focus on a lifeworld perspective to understand the real essence of individuals' experiences of their first encounter with pre-hospital emergency care services.

Methods of data collection: Unstructured interviews with people who have actually experienced this situation. An unstructured interview allows the researchers to explore the uniqueness of the event with each individual participant in depth without being constrained by predetermined questions/topics.

Key concepts: The researchers attempted to 'bridle' their preconceptions (bracketing) to avoid influencing the findings. Unstructured interviews increase opportunities to recognise emergent multiple realities.

Practical considerations: Elmqvist et al. identify that the interviews were extensive and varied in length between 45 and 155 minutes. This can be a challenge in analysis in terms of ensuring fair representation of each individual's contribution.

Verdict on Elmqvist et al.'s research – phenomenology or not?

YES

Grounded theory

Grounded theory has its roots in sociology (in particular the sociological perspective of symbolic interactionism) and is focussed on developing theory related to social processes grounded in the data obtained from study participants (Box 7.5). Glaser and Strauss (1967) developed an approach to grounded theory which has influenced many studies in healthcare and, over the years, different perspectives on grounded theory have emerged. Morse et al. (2009) state:

As with all qualitative methods – and perhaps all research methods – the method cannot be used in a 'cookbook' or formulaic way. Every application, every time grounded theory is used, it requires adaptation in particular ways as demanded by the research question, situation, and participants for whom the research is being conducted. But grounded theory is not necessarily a collection of strategies. It is primarily a particular way of thinking about data. (2009: 14)

Box 7.5 Characteristics of grounded theory

Tradition sociology

Focus theory generation; to enable theories to emerge from the data through processes of constant comparison; exploration of social processes and explaining human behaviour

Common methods of data collection in-depth interviews (frequently unstructured); observation; study of documents, diaries, other records; blogs

Key concepts keeping an open mind; constant comparative method; development of emergent theory; theoretical sampling; data saturation; coding and categorisation in analysis

Practical considerations difficulties of approaching the research without any preconceived ideas; many variations to the original concept of grounded theory; making
sure that emergent theories are 'grounded' in the data

N.B. You may not find all of these characteristics in every grounded theory research
study

Morse et al. identify that researchers have frequently adapted this methodology
selecting only some elements of the theory rather than adopting a totally grounded
theory approach within their study. Even Glaser and Strauss themselves had a
parting of the ways and constructed distinct versions of grounded theory as they
could not agree on certain elements. So you will come across several variations of
grounded theory in your reading.

In grounded theory the processes of analysis are central to this approach as the
interpretation of the data is a key activity. Analysis is **iterative** and **inductive**
using processes of **constant comparison** of data so that as concepts emerge they
are constantly compared to new data until no new concepts and/or theories emerge
(Glaser and Strauss 1967).

Challenges in grounded theory research

- **Theoretical sampling** is a core strategy in grounded theory that facilitates
effective processes of constant comparison. The researcher does not know in
advance who will be in their sample as it is only when the concepts and theories
emerge that the researcher can make decisions as to whom or what will be the
most appropriate sample to include next. This is a challenge in grounded theory
studies as researchers are not able to identify sample characteristics before the
study commences as these decisions will depend on emergent data. This can be
problematic when approaching a Research Ethics Committee (REC) or funding
body as this information will not be available at the start of the study.

- **Theoretical saturation** should determine the end of data collection (Glaser
1992). This is when no new data emerges and the constant comparison activities
only reinforce existing interpretations. Hence the size of sample required for the
study is unknown at the start of the project which, again, can be of concern to
RECs or funders.

- Having an 'open mind'. Researchers should not have any preconceived ideas
or expectations as to what they might find in the study before it starts. Taken
to the extreme, this prohibits reviewing the literature before developing and
undertaking the research. This decision is not without risk as if the researcher is
unaware of similar studies in the same field as they have not reviewed existing
literature, there could be unnecessary duplication of research which is neither
practical or ethical (Denscombe 2003).

These challenges all require the researcher to make methodological decisions.
Sometimes these decisions have to be based on practicalities. For example, if the
study has to be submitted to an REC, then the background to the research will

need to be presented and this will more than likely require the researcher to consult existing literature. These types of issues may be why some researchers using grounded theory only adopt part of the approach to accommodate their needs, rather than engaging in the whole process.

An example of a grounded theory study in paramedic practice

Campeau (2009) undertook a piece of research designed to increase understanding of how paramedics actually manage situations on-scene. He set out 'to generate a substantive theory of paramedic scene management practice' (2009: 213). He wanted to explore how paramedics take control of their working environments and how they adapt them to provide emergency healthcare.

Campeau decided to adopt a grounded theory approach using semi-structured interviews which were audio-recorded and transcribed prior to analysis. In total, 24 paramedics were involved:

- 14 male, 10 female

- 10 from urban areas, 9 from suburban areas and 5 from rural areas

- 6 were novice level practitioners; 7 were experienced practitioners; and 11 were deemed to be experts.

Campeau identifies that he carried out three rounds of interviews but it is not clear in the paper whether, and if so how, he used theoretical sampling. However, this is a good point to note. Just because activities are not described in a publication, it does not mean we can assume that they were not done. All that can be said in an appraisal is that these issues were not mentioned. Although not making specific reference to theoretical sampling, Campeau does refer to constant comparison of data between each round of interviews in order to check the emerging theories against new data.

Ultimately, Campeau developed the first 'formal theory of paramedic scene management' (2009: 213) known as the Space Control Theory. The theory comprises five categories pertaining to social processes on-scene:

- establishing a safety zone

- reducing uncertainty through social relations

- controlling the trajectory of the scene

- temporality at the scene

- collateral monitoring.

Through this research (Box 7.6), Campeau argues that defining this theory, which is grounded in paramedics' views and experiences, will help to improve understanding of other healthcare professionals as to what actually happens on-scene. He believes this theory will be useful for enhancing educational developments for paramedics and student paramedics by providing a theory of practice. Campeau would like to see the development of more theories that examine paramedic practice from a broader perspective than just patient assessment and intervention (2008).

Box 7.6 Evidence of characteristics relevant to grounded theory in Campeau's (2008) study

Focus: Campeau stated as an objective for the research that he wanted to generate a theory, in this case, to explain paramedic scene management.

Methods of data collection: Campeau uses semi-structured interviews to gather the data on this occasion. You could also consider using observation in this situation. This could add another dimension to the data by actually observing how paramedics engage in scene management.

Key concepts: Data collection and analysis occurred simultaneously. Campeau adopted an approach of constant comparison of data whereby as ideas and concepts emerged he would check these against new data that he was collecting. This is why he had three rounds of interviews.

Practical considerations: Demonstrating to readers that theories have emerged from the data can be challenging. Detailed description of the processes of constant comparison during the stages of analysis is essential. A reflexive journal and careful documentation of the audit trail can be useful in providing this evidence.

Verdict on Campeau's research – grounded theory or not?

YES

Generic qualitative research

Not all qualitative research 'fits' the approaches that have been discussed so far and researchers should not be pressured into following a research approach if it is not suited to the study's aim(s). Some of the published qualitative research in pre-hospital care emphasises the exploration of clinical issues but does not necessarily align with any specific qualitative research approach (Box 7.7).

Box 7.7 Characteristics of generic qualitative research

Tradition influenced by various approaches; traditions, methods

Focus study of human experience; views/opinions, perceptions; understanding

Common methods of data collection: interviews; open ended surveys; focus groups; observation; documents; photos; diaries; blogs

Key concepts description of strategies for rigour; alignment of methods and methodology; flexibility; purpose of the study does not 'fit' other established research approaches

Practical considerations need to provide in-depth details about methodological decision making and processes to ensure rigour; avoid methodological slurring

N.B. These characteristics will vary according to the selected research approaches within the study

As we have seen with other research approaches, although there may be significant variations within the same approach, readers may have an expectation of what structure or processes could be involved in research aligned with an established methodology. With generic qualitative research these preconceptions do not exist as the design could include a combination of a variety of qualitative methods.

Caelli et al. acknowledge the need for generic qualitative research but they are concerned about the quality of this work:

> *We define generic qualitative research as that which is not guided by an explicit or established set of philosophic assumptions in the form of one of the known qualitative methodologies...There is a need and a place for generic qualitative research – the question is how to do it well.* (2003: 2)

They suggest four areas that should be included when writing accounts of qualitative research so that the reader can make their own evaluations of quality:

1   Theoretical positioning of the researcher. This refers to the reasons that the researcher wants to do the research, their motivations, background, interests, and existing beliefs.

2   Congruence between methodology and methods. There needs to be a fit between methods and methodology. The methodology is about the philosophical underpinnings of the research. The methods need to be appropriate for the research approach with sufficient detail given to demonstrate their effective use. Caelli et al. warn that generic qualitative research should not become an unstructured approach where researchers just borrow elements of recognised research approaches and then try and patch them all together (sometimes referred to as 'method slurring'). There needs to be a good fit between methods and research approach.

3   Strategies to establish rigour. These are complex and as we saw in Chapter 6 there is no consensus as to the most appropriate processes to achieve this in qualitative research. However, qualitative research must be rigorous and qualitative researchers need to keep developing in this area in order to ensure their research is credible.

4   The analytic lens through which the data are examined. This refers to how researchers look at the data and what informs their approach to making sense of the data.

At first glance, there may seem to be some overlap between points 1 and 4, but Caelli et al. (2003: 8) clarify that: 'While theoretical positioning was about the researcher and his or her motives for pursuing a particular area of inquiry, the analytic lens is about how the researcher engages with his or her data'.

In their conclusions, Caelli et al. indicate that generic qualitative research is here to stay and they identify a need for greater knowledge and an increased evidence base to support this research approach.

An example of a generic qualitative research study in paramedic practice

There are several studies that have been undertaken in pre-hospital emergency care that do not identify specific affiliation to any particular research approach. A mixed-method study by Cooper et al. (2007) explored the role of the emergency care practitioner (ECP) by adopting a generic qualitative approach to the qualitative components of the study.

The study was presented in two papers: one focussing on the qualitative components and the other on the quantitative elements. The aim of the study was 'to develop an overview of the current ECP role by identifying instances and hindrances to collaboration and from this to develop a model of collaboration in unscheduled care' (2007: 625).

The qualitative components comprised observation (field-notes were documented) and interviews with 24 ECPs (nurses and paramedics). In addition interviews were carried out with 21 stakeholders from a variety of professional backgrounds including doctors, nurses, paramedics, social services, trust managers, practice managers and care home managers.

The interviews were semi-structured and explored topics around the ECP role and collaborative working.

The authors describe the process of analysis in detail and link this to processes of triangulation of data which Cooper and Endacott (2007) advocate should be considered to establish rigour within generic qualitative research. Cooper et al.'s findings from systematic and rigorous analysis include identification of three major themes:

- ECP role

- cultural perspectives

- education and training.

Cooper et al. take the opportunity in the paper to map their study against Caelli et al.'s four quality criteria by:

1 describing the research teams' background and interests and by declaring preconceived ideas

2 describing the methods and linking them to methodology

3 outlining their actions to improve rigour e.g.:
   ○ keeping an audit trail
   ○ independent analysis of the interview transcripts between the two researchers
   ○ having a respondent validation event to discuss what had emerged from the analysis
   ○ use of triangulation by using a number of different data sources

4 describing how they engaged with the data – the analytical lens.

This paper provides an impressive account of the application of key quality criteria to generic qualitative research. However, one point to consider is that this description took over half of the discussion section, which whilst commendable may not always be possible depending on the word limit of the publication. Nonetheless this is the type of information that needs to be included within the audit trail in case researchers are approached for further details about their research study.

From this type of research (Box 7.8), Cooper et al. produced a model of collaborative practice involving ECPs and they made several recommendations for service developments which could benefit patient care.

Box 7.8 Evidence of characteristics relevant to generic qualitative research in Cooper et al.'s (2007) study

Focus: Cooper et al. wanted to find out more about participants' experiences and understanding of the ECP role, and their views about the contribution of ECPs to unscheduled healthcare provision.

Methods of data collection: In the qualitative component of the study, Cooper et al. used semi-structured interviews lasting 20–30 minutes with a variety of different professionals; plus periods of observation with ECPs. Use of different sources of data is one example of triangulation (see Chapter 6).

Key concepts: Clearly the aims of the study required a flexible research approach. Cooper et al. demonstrate how the methods align with the research approach and show a good 'fit' between them. They provide an excellent account of how they address Caelli et al.'s four quality criteria that we looked at earlier in this chapter.

Practical considerations: Need to make sure that generic qualitative research is not just a pick and mix of unlinked methods (method slurring). Providing a description of methodological decision making is time consuming and difficult to fit in to a published paper with word restrictions – you need to get a balance between description of activities to enhance rigour and presentation of research findings.

Verdict on Cooper et al.'s research – generic qualitative research or not?

YES

Conclusion

There are many different research approaches within qualitative research; it is not a case of 'one size fits all'. The decision as to which approach to use for what study should be based on identification of the approach that is most appropriate to explore the topic area, and which gives the best chance of answering the research question(s). Researchers and those critiquing research need to be fully informed about the possible options and they should understand the strengths and limitations of the chosen approach.

This chapter introduces four possible approaches, but there are many more. Hopefully it has emphasised that not all qualitative research is the same and neither do all the research approaches have the same purpose. However, all qualitative research must be undertaken in a systematic, rigorous way to ensure that it maintains its place as a recognised contributor to scientific endeavour and knowledge development.

References

Caelli, K., Ray, L. and Mill, J. (2003) 'Clear as mud': toward greater clarity in generic qualitative research. *International Journal of Qualitative Methods* 2(2): 1–13.

Campeau, A. (2008) Professionalism: why paramedics require 'Theories-of-Practice'. *Journal of Emergency Primary Healthcare* 6(2): Article 990296

Campeau, A. (2009) Introduction to the 'space-control theory of paramedic scene management'. *Emergency Medical Journal* 26(3): 213–216.

Cooper, S. and Endacott, R. (2007) Generic qualitative research: a design for qualitative research in emergency care? *Emergency Medical Journal* 24(12): 816–819.

Cooper, S., O' Carroll, J., Jenkin, A. and Badger, B. (2007) Collaborative practices in unscheduled emergency care: role and impact of the emergency care practitioner: qualitative and summative findings. *Emergency Medical Journal* 24(9): 624–629.

Creswell, J.W. (2007) *Qualitative Inquiry and Research Design: Choosing Among Five Approaches* (2nd edn). Thousand Oaks, CA: Sage Publications.

Denscombe, M. (2003) *The Good Research Guide* (2nd edn). Maidenhead: Open University Press.

Elmqvist, C., Fridlund, B. and Ekebergh, M. (2008) More than medical treatment: the patient's first encounter with prehospital emergency care. *International Emergency Nursing* 16(3): 185–192.

Flood, A. (2010) Understanding phenomenology. *Nurse Researcher* 17(2): 7–15.

Giorgi, A. (1997) The theory, practice, and evaluation of the phenomenological method as a qualitative research procedure. *Journal of Phenomenological Psychology* 28(2): 235–261.

Glaser, B.G. (1992) *The Basics of Grounded Theory Analysis: Emergence vs. Forcing*. Mill Valley, CA: Sociology Press.

Glaser, B.G. and Strauss, A.L. (1967) *The Discovery of Grounded Theory*. New York: Aldine.

Hammersley, M. and Atkinson, P. (1983) *Ethnography: Principles in Practice*. London: Routledge.

Heidegger, M. (1962) *Being and Time*. Oxford: Basil Blackwell.

Lincoln, Y.S. and Guba, E.G. (1985) *Naturalistic Inquiry*. Beverly Hills, CA: Sage Publications.

Lofland, J. (1976) *Doing Social Life: The Qualitative Study of Human Interaction in Natural Settings*. New York: John Wiley.

Manning, P.K. and Van Maanen, J. (eds) (1978) *Policing: A View from the Streets*. Santa Monica, CA: Goodyear.

Morse, J.M., Stern, P.N., Corbin, J. Bowers, B., Charmaz, K. and Clarke, A.E. (2009) *Developing Grounded Theory: The Second Generation*. Walnut Creek, CA: Left Coast Press.

Palmer, C.E. (1983) Trauma Junkies and Street Work: occupational behaviours of paramedics and emergency medical technicians. *Journal of Contemporary Ethnography* 12(2): 162–183.

Parahoo, K. (2006) *Nursing Research: Principles, Process and Issues* (2nd edn). Basingstoke: Palgrave Macmillan.

8 Quantitative research in paramedic practice: an overview

Jayne Cutter

Learning outcomes for the chapter

By the end of this chapter the reader should be able to:

1   Understand how a suitable quantitative research question is formulated

2   Understand how a sample representative of the population is identified

3   Understand how a research approach most appropriate to address the research question is decided on

4   Consider the suitability of simple descriptive and inferential statistical tests for data analysis

Keywords
quantitative
reliability
sampling rigour
statistics
validity

Introduction

This chapter aims to provide a broad overview of quantitative research starting at the point of deciding a research project will be undertaken through to data analysis and all important stages in between. It is not designed to be a complete 'how to' guide on undertaking quantitative research, rather it is a basic guide to understanding the process that will allow you to more out of reading quantitative research studies and hopefully enable you to make your first foray into conducting your own research projects.

The stages of research to be discussed in the following chapters will offer a systematic approach to quantitative research that will guide you through the research process from idea to output (Figure 8.1).

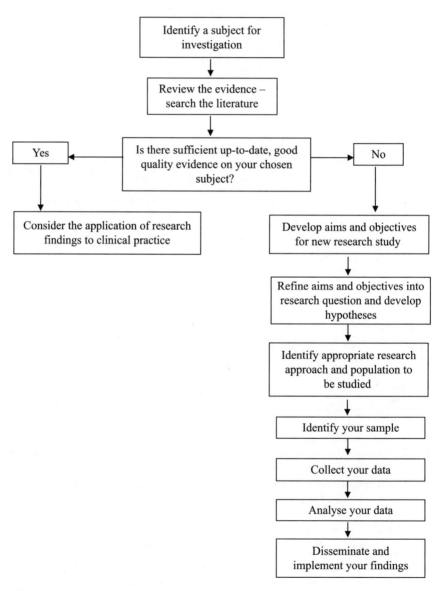

Figure 8.1 Stages in the quantitative research process

Research questions: hypothesis and null hypothesis

The first stage in designing a research project is to decide on a subject of interest that requires investigation, either because little or no research exists in the field or more likely because the available research is out of date, incomplete or simply bears further investigation. The aims and objectives of the study will identify what the researcher is trying to achieve and provide a collection of goals to which the researcher will aspire. However, these aims and objectives may be vague and need to be focussed. To do this a research question is posed.

The origin of the research question is often found in previous studies and may be generated following a review of the literature. The research question in a quantitative study will frequently begin with 'do/does', 'what is' or 'how many' rather than 'how' or 'why' (Box 8.1).

Box 8.1 An example of a research question

In 2009 a study with two objectives was published in *Prehospital Emergency Care*. Firstly, to determine emergency medical technicians' (EMS) opinions on participation in disease and injury prevention and secondly to determine the proportion of EMS professionals who had done so. These objectives were refined into the following research question:
'Do EMS professionals think they should participate in disease prevention?'
(Lerner et al. 2009).

Some researchers will endeavour to make predictions about the expected outcome of a study before even beginning to collect data. These predictions will relate to the expectation that a relationship between variables will be established (a hypothesis) or that no relationship will be established (a null hypothesis). The purpose of the study will then be to accept or reject the hypothesis (or null hypothesis), see Box 8.2.

Box 8.2 An example of a hypothesis

Chen and Hsiao (2008) hypothesised that in simulated pre-hospital arrests in children the use of laryngeal mask airway (LMA) would result in a shorter time to effective ventilation than endotracheal tubes when used by emergency medical services personnel.
They also hypothesised that fewer complications would result from using LMA. The subsequent research study accepted both hypotheses.

Quantitative approaches to designing research studies

Having posed the research question, and identified the hypothesis (or null hypothesis), an appropriate research approach must be identified. Quantitative research is most suited to exploring variables that can be measured and relationships between variables are examined objectively either statistically or numerically to provide an answer to the question. A variable is 'an attribute that varies, that is, takes on different values (e.g. body temperature, heart rate)' (Polit and Beck 2008: 768) and may be classed as dependent or independent. A dependent variable will be influenced or depend on another variable (the *independent variable*), see Box 8.3.

Box 8.3 Dependent and independent variables

Siriwardena et al. (2009) set out to investigate whether cannulation technique and inappropriate cannulation by paramedics (the dependent variables) were influenced by an educational intervention (the independent variable).

Quantitative research methods include either *non-experimental* or experimental studies (Bowling 2009).

Non-experimental methods include:

- surveys
- descriptive studies
- analytical studies
- cross-sectional studies
- *prospective studies*
- secondary analysis.

Experimental methods include:

- experiments e.g. laboratory
- *randomised controlled trials (RCTs)*
- *quasi-experiments*
- explanatory surveys
- observational studies.

A non-experimental study establishes only associations between variables while an experiment establishes causality. These will be discussed in more detail in Chapter 9.

Sampling

A population is the entire group of people in which a researcher is interested, for example all paramedics in the UK, or all patients who have suffered a myocardial infarction in Wales during 2011. In general, quantitative researchers will endeavour to include as many participants as possible in their studies as the more participants included, the more the findings can be generalised to the total population studied. Including an entire population in a research project is usually prohibitive in terms of cost or access. Therefore, researchers need to select a **subset** of the population that can be considered representative of the whole for inclusion in the study.

This subset of the population is known as the sample and its characteristics must closely approximate the characteristics of the population, for example the same gender or age distribution. Sampling is the process by which a sample is selected. Sampling designs are considered either as **probability sampling** in which the sample is selected randomly or **non-probability sampling** in which the sample is selected by non randomised means.

Characteristics of probability sampling

- Everyone within a population has an equal chance of being selected increasing the likelihood that the sample is representative of the population.

- Selection is random; therefore, no bias is possible. This adds to the credibility of probability sampling.

- Probability sampling is often impractical unless the population is narrowly defined e.g. patients within a narrow age range suffering from the same medical condition.

Characteristics of non-probability sampling

- The strength of non-probability sampling lies in its practicality particularly when the population is not narrowly defined e.g. all paramedics in the UK.

- A non-probability sample may not be representative of the population.

- A non-probability sample cannot be considered free of bias.

Types of probability sampling

Probability sampling utilises a sampling frame or a list of potential participants and includes:

- **Simple random sampling** – each potential participant is allocated a number and numbers selected randomly. Each number has an equal chance of being drawn 'out of the hat'. Random number tables or computer packages that generate random number sequences can be used to simplify the process.

- **Systematic random sampling** – participants are chosen at intervals from a list; for example every tenth person.

- **Stratified random sampling** – the target population is divided into strata or divisions according to predetermined characteristics, e.g. age, height or weight before implementing simple or systematic random sampling.

- **Cluster random sampling** – this relies on the fact that some study populations can be organised into clusters or groups of similar entities – houses in a street, doctors in a hospital. Cluster sampling involves several stages. If a researcher wanted to consider patients sustaining fractured neck of femur within one city, firstly he would identify the city, then the NHS trust, then the hospital accepting trauma patients, then the relevant orthopaedic ward and finally the patients.

Types of non-probability sampling

Non-probability sampling is common in health service research. The following types of non-probability sampling are frequently used:

- **Convenience sampling** – this entails approaching the most convenient people, often because they are known to the researcher or the researcher has easy access to them. Market research where pedestrians are stopped in the street, lecturers who involve their students in a study, paramedics surveying patients for whom they have provided care utilise convenience sampling.

- **Snowball sampling** – is a form of convenience sampling where early participants recommend others that they think may be suitable participants.

- **Quota sampling** – this can be considered similar to stratified sampling in that certain characteristics within a sample, religion or ethnicity for example, are sought. This means that where the views of one group may be significantly different to another, a suitable sample can be identified which represents the proportion in which each group is represented in society. For example, African–Caribbean males may experience more racial abuse than white males. Therefore in a study which seeks to examine the frequency of racial incidents in an inner city school, an over-representation of white males will not provide accurate data. Therefore, quota sampling would be appropriate to identify the correct proportion of white to African–Caribbean males.

- **Purposive sampling** – this relies on the researcher's belief that they know the population and relies on the researcher's judgements on their suitability for inclusion. However, there is a degree of subjectivity here that may compromise the rigour of the study.

If the sample is not representative of the population, the external and construct validity will be compromised and the study's findings may not be considered valid. According to Bowling (2005) two types of sampling error exist: systematic error where sampling is carried out incorrectly and random error where an unusually unrepresentative sample is chosen. The result of sampling error when testing a hypothesis could be that either a true hypothesis is rejected (Type 1 error), or a null hypothesis is accepted (Type 2 error).

Data collection methods

A variety of collection tools are used to collect data in quantitative studies. According to Parahoo, these include questionnaires, observations schedules, scales and instruments but all are 'predetermined, structured and standardised' (2006: 55). In experimental research, physiological and mechanical measurement tools are often used according to the measurements required. It is beyond the scope of this chapter to describe these; however, in both experimental and descriptive studies, two data collection methods are frequently used – direct observation and surveys.

Observation

Direct observation is often a suitable method of data collection where participants may not report behaviour or events accurately and is particularly suitable for observing non-verbal behaviour where self-reported data may not accurately capture true behaviour due to embarrassment, fear of censure or where the research subjects cannot articulate their viewpoints, for example those who may be unconscious, distressed or confused, and is frequently used in descriptive research. Checklists or rating scales may be used to record observations. Using a standardised checklist means that multiple observers can be used to speed up data collection while ensuring that the phenomena are observed and recorded in the same way. The researcher becomes the measuring instrument but recording equipment can be useful in enhancing the researcher's observation skills and increasing continuity where several researchers are used to collect data. Recording also means that more than one person can view the recording thereby minimising bias. However, despite the availability of recording equipment and checklists the role of observer can be difficult (see Chapter 9).

Survey

One of the most common data collection methods used in descriptive quantitative research is the survey. Surveys are also useful in descriptive studies although many of us are familiar with surveys from our everyday lives in the form of satisfaction surveys, opinion polls, the national census carried out every ten years in the UK and market research. Surveys rely on self-reported data, that is, individuals answering a series of questions posed by the researcher either face-to-face or in the absence of the investigator often via the mail or internet. Surveys are useful when a researcher wishes to consider knowledge, behaviour and attitudes. Structured questions can be used to collect unambiguous data that lends itself well to data analysis using computerised statistical packages and are therefore suited to areas where little research exists. Not only are surveys useful to capture data on events that have already happened, but can also be used to collect information on what may or may not happen in the future.

Survey questions do not ask for in-depth answers but rely on a series of brief predetermined responses – 'yes/no' 'male/female' etc. – to collect extensive but, some would argue, rather superficial data. Having said that, more detailed responses can be encouraged by the use of scales, commonly called *Likert scales*, in which a range of potential responses is provided (see Box 8.4) for example, 'excellent, very good, good, satisfactory, poor'. These are commonly used in studies that measure attitude.

Box 8.4 Example of a study using a Likert scale

Rajabali et al. (2008) utilised a four point Likert scale to evaluate attitudes and perceptions of key clinical stakeholders regarding out-of-hours diagnosis and treatment of myocardial infarction patients.

Surveys utilise a number of approaches to collect data. Face-to-face interviews involve an interviewer meeting with participant to ask a series of questions. This is a labour intensive strategy which may require specific training for the interviewer but the benefit is that response rates in face-to-face interviews tend to be high. Telephone interviews also rely on an interviewer asking questions of the participants but without the expense and labour intensive input required in face-to-face interviews. They are most suited to relatively short interviews but response rates will be lower than with face-to-face interviews as those who may consider it impolite to turn away from an interviewer may be less reluctant to hang up on a telephone call. They may be inconvenient for those with hearing difficulties or those without phones who will not be able to be accessed and therefore a sample may be unrepresentative of the general population. Electronic surveys are increasingly used for research purposes and free online software such as SurveyMonkey are easily accessible. Electronic surveys are simple and relatively cheap to administer and can reach a large target audience but this audience is limited to those with internet access and some groups of the population, particularly the older adult and those in low socio-economic groups where internet access may be difficult could be excluded. It is possible that internet security systems may block the messages so that the intended recipients do not receive the questionnaire. Incompatibility between operating systems such as Apple and Microsoft may also reduce the potential sample size.

Market research often utilises face-to-face, telephone and electronic interviews. However, more common in healthcare research is the use of postal questionnaires. These allow distribution to a large number of geographically spread participants easily. Postal questionnaires minimise the social desirability response where respondents may be influenced in their responses by consideration of how their answer may affect or be judged by the interviewer and therefore it is possible they may be more honest in their responses. The social desirability response could therefore introduce bias into the survey.

Rigour in quantitative research

The concept of rigour in research relates to the strength of the design, the amount of bias and the degree of control over extraneous variables. In quantitative research it is discussed in terms of validity and reliability.

Validity

It is important that a measurement tool measures what it purports to measure. Validity is the extent to which the data collection tool measures what it is intended to measure:

- **Content validity** is where each item on a questionnaire or interview schedule is examined for relevance and is inevitably, to some extent, based on the judgement of practitioners and academics. One element of content validity is face validity which refers to whether the data collection tool looks as if it measures the construct under question. An instrument can be said to have face validity if one can determine what is being measured by looking at the tool.

- **Criterion-related validity** relates to how well a new instrument compares with other tried and tested measures such as a different questionnaire or direct observation. The validity of a new instrument is difficult to establish, agreement is often reached concerning the relative validity of frequently used instruments and where existing data collection tools are available, they should be used in preference to designing a new un-validated instrument.

- **Construct validity** also referred to as measurement validity, refers to whether the questionnaire yields results that confirm statistical relationships derived from existing theory and so relates to assumptions made on theoretical knowledge (Oppenheim 1992).

- **Ecological validity** is the extent to which findings are applicable to participants' natural social settings. However, it has been suggested that the falseness of having to complete a questionnaire and the social desirability response could mean that ecological validity is compromised (Bryman 2008).

- **Internal validity** relates to the degree to which cause and effect can be demonstrated and refers to the extent to which changes in the dependent variable can be attributed to changes in the independent variable. Experiments possess a high degree of internal validity because variables can be manipulated to rule out alternative explanations for the results. *Randomisation* further increases internal validity.

- **External validity** or the degree to which the behaviour and opinions of the sample population are representative of the wider population and represents the extent to which the findings of a study can be generalised to other settings. External validity will be increased but not guaranteed by a large sample and compromised by a low response rate.

Reliability

Reliability is the degree of consistency with which a measurement tool measures what it is designed to measure. It relates to both the instrument of data collection, i.e. the questionnaire, and the conditions under which it is administered and can be measured by its level of purity, consistency and accuracy. Reliability may be considered as having two aspects – external and internal reliability.

- **External reliability** or stability represents consistency over time. To an extent the same measurement tool, e.g. questionnaire, should provide the same information whenever it is administered within the same population. However, it must be recognised that traits and opinions change over time and experiences, memory and boredom with repetition may alter the participant's responses and lack of correlation may not necessarily be due to an unreliable research instrument. Researchers may evaluate the stability of an instrument by evaluating the **test-retest reliability** which involves using the same data collection instrument twice and comparing the results. A statistic known as the **reliability coefficient** may be employed to indicate the degree of reliability by describing the strength of the relationship between variables. A perfect relationship is indicated by a correlation coefficient of 1.00.

- **Internal reliability** or consistency relates to whether a scale is comprised of consistent indicators (Bryman 2008) and the extent to which the questions within a scale measure each phenomenon being studied can be measured using a statistic known as **Cronbach's alpha** in which a score of 0 to 1.00 indicates the degree of **internal consistency**.

Where more than one observer is involved in the data collection process, it is important that each agrees with the evaluation or description of the event to minimise measurement errors. **Interrator reliability** can be measured by two or more researchers participating in an observation simultaneously and comparing their findings. It could be assumed that a high level of agreement confers high interrator reliability. However, agreement may happen by coincidence and so a statistic known as **Cohen's kappa** can be used to adjust for chance. The value of Cohen's kappa is measured between 0 and 1.00 and a level of 0.6 or above would be considered acceptable (Polit and Beck 2008).

Whereas use of a previously used measurement tool may improve validity, there is no guarantee that doing this will enhance reliability as reliability relates not only to the instrument but the conditions under which it is administered. Hence a questionnaire administered to patients experiencing pre-hospital care may not be suitable for those in a long-term hospital.

Statistical concepts

Measurement

Quantitative research examines relationships between variables numerically or statistically. The mere mention of statistics can elicit cries of horror from those who 'don't like numbers'. However, statistics can be used effectively to clearly present research findings and a deep understanding of intricate mathematical concepts is not required.

The complexity of the statistics presented will depend on the type of measurement used. **Nominal measurement** is the lowest form of measurement and relates to categories that can be named and assigned a simple numerical code, for example male/female where male may be assigned the number 1 and female the number 2. Nominal categories must be mutually exclusive and bear some relation to each other – we are all biologically either male or female. An unsuitable combination of categories would be paramedic/blood group A/female because some participants may fit into two or more of these categories.

Ordinal measurement allows sorting of data based on a ranking system. Ordinal measurement implies some degree of order, for example average, good and excellent but while order is apparent, the difference between each category is not quantifiable. Although you can assign numbers to each category, for example average = 1, good = 2, excellent = 3, these numbers do not quantify any difference between the categories, i.e. excellent is not three times better than average. Nominal and ordinal data are described as *categorical data*.

Interval measurement permits rank ordering of data where a regular interval is apparent between the categories, for example patients' temperature recordings of 36°C, 37°C, 38°C and 39°C where each successive temperature measurement is 1°C higher than the previous one. However, interval measurements do not have an absolute zero.

Ratio measurements have an absolute zero. Examination marks can be considered as ratio data because a mark of zero can and occasionally does occur. It is possible to say that a student achieving a mark of 100% had a score of ten times that of a student awarded 10% whereas these comparisons are not possible with interval data. You cannot, for example say that a person with a temperature of 35°C is 5% colder than someone whose temperature is 40°C as a body temperature of zero is impossible in a living patient. Interval and ratio data are described as *continuous data*.

Descriptive statistics

Descriptive statistics are used to describe data. In its simplest form, descriptive statistics will tell us the frequency or number of responses to any particular question and is expressed as a number (n) or percentage and even with this simple measure, information on a given variable emerges from the data (Box 8.5).

Box 8.5 An example of a study using descriptive statistics

Jones et al. (2008) investigated whether there was any continuity or plan in the use of pre-hospital dressings on soft tissue trauma. All the findings were presented as frequencies e.g. 27% of UK ambulance services had a specific wound management policy; 27% used Steristrips; 40% used gauze swabs etc.

From these simple descriptive statistics, the authors were able to conclude that there is no national standard protocol for wound management in the UK ambulance service and could subsequently recommend a service improvement, namely, that a simple wound management protocol is developed.

Sometimes, we are interested in an average or measure of *central tendency* rather than an absolute number. In statistics, we refer to three types of average. To illustrate these, let us consider a group of patients and categorise them according to their age in years, where we have a distribution of ages as follows:

$$12, 36, 55, 68, 75, 75, 75, 69, 57, 40, 10$$

The **mode** is the most frequently occurring value in a distribution. In this example, the most frequently occurring age, i.e. the mode, is 75.

Now let us consider these patients again. The **median** is the value below and above which an equal number of cases occur. To calculate this, the numbers are first arranged in ascending order:

$$10, 12, 36, 40, 55, 57, 68, 69, 75, 75, 75$$

In these patients, the median is 57 as five ages appear below and five appear above.

The **mean** is the sum of all values divided by the number of values in your dataset

$$\frac{12 + 36 + 55 + 68 + 75 + 75 + 75 + 69 + 57 + 40 + 10}{11} = 52$$

The **range** is the highest minus the lowest score. In our example, this would be:

$$75 - 10 = 65$$

Graphical representation of distribution

Distributions can also be organised visually. This allows us to look for patterns in the data. Figure 8.2 is a normal distribution curve or bell-shaped curve and represents a distribution of ages arranged symmetrically where the highest frequency

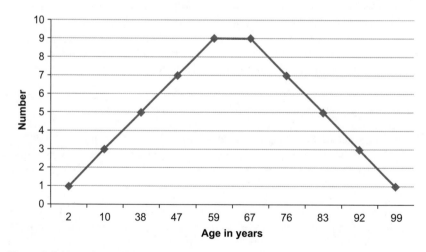

Figure 8.2 Normal distribution

of ages were distributed near the midpoint and exceptionally low or high ages at each extreme.

In a situation where a large number of young patients are seen and plotted on a graph, the highest density of ages is clustered towards the lower end of the age range and the resulting graph is said to have a *positive skew* where the long tail of the graph is directed in positive direction (Figure 8.3).

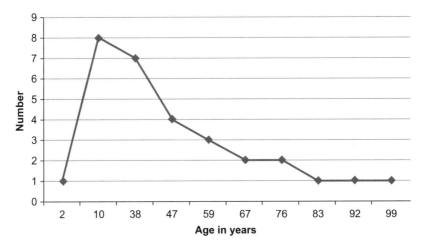

Figure 8.3 Positive skew

Now imagine that most of the patients seen are elderly: the largest frequency of ages would be seen at the higher end and the graph would now be said to have a *negative skew* (Figure 8.4).

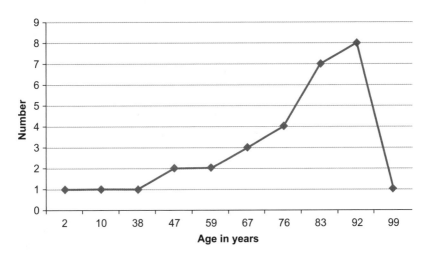

Figure 8.4 Negative skew

Inferential statistics

As useful as descriptive statistics are, they only describe single variables. *Inferential statistics* help us explore relationships between variables from which we can make inferences from the sample population to the general population. A range of statistical tests is available to help us explore relationships in data. Choice of test depends on whether:

- data are categorical or continuous
- data are normally distributed.

Where data are normally distributed parametric tests can be used whereas non-parametric tests must be used where data are not normally distributed. Normally distributed data are predictable: values will always be distributed in a certain pattern (Figure 8.2). Therefore, statistical tests applied to normally distributed data carry with them a high degree of certainty. Data that are not distributed normally lack this predictability and therefore non-parametric tests lack the certainty of parametric tests and are therefore considered less rigorous.

It is beyond the scope of this chapter to describe in detail the range of statistical tests. However, common tests for exploring relationships between categorical data include the *Chi-square* and *Fisher's exact tests*. Continuous data are frequently explored using tests such as the *Mann-Whitney U test*, *Kruskal-Wallis test* (non-parametric) and one and two tailed t-tests (parametric). However, regardless of the tests applied, one factor stands out as being of paramount importance in inferential statistics, i.e. that of significance.

Significance testing

Significance testing is a method by which researchers can identify whether a relationship truly exists between variables. Significance is based on percentages and assumes that we can never be 100% certain of our findings. We must therefore apply criteria that describe how certain we are. Typically, the criteria we apply are 95% (most commonly) or 99% which assume that we are either 95% or 99% confident of our findings or described another way, only 5% or 1% of our findings occurred by chance. We then have significance levels of 0.05 (5%) or 0.01 (1%). Significance is expressed by the letter p which represents the probability that the null hypothesis is true. A relationship is said to be statistically significance if $p < 0.05$ or $p < 0.01$ depending on the criterion that we apply i.e. there is less than 5% or 1% probability that this relationship occurred by chance (Box 8.6).

> **Box 8.6** An example of a study with statistical significance
>
> Rajabali et al. (2008) explored the attitudes and perceptions of key stakeholders regarding out of hours diagnosis and treatment of myocardial infarction. An attitude scale was used to collect data.

Results were expressed as percentages of respondents who strongly agreed/agreed/disagreed/strongly disagreed with a list of statements.

Using inferential statistics, the authors were able to explore different relationships e.g. the level of agreement between professions on various treatment protocols. P values were calculated to identify whether these relationships occurred by chance or were statistically significant. For example, 50%–51% of cardiologists and emergency physicians compared to 78%–81% paramedics or emergency nurses felt that signed informed consent was necessary before administering in-hospital fibrinolysis.

The difference between these groups was statistically significant ($p < 0.005$). However, no statisticaly significance was found between the groups in relation to signed informed consent and pre-hospital administration of fibrinolysis ($p = 0.13$).

Another way of expressing significance is by considering the *confidence interval* (CI). A confidence interval is the estimated range of values that contains the true value at a level we consider a relationship significant, usually 95% or 99%. Rather than have a single absolute value, a confidence interval describes a margin of error. Again, confidence intervals are expressed as percentages. A confidence interval of 95% (CI 95%) offers two values between which we can be 95% confident that the true value lies (Box 8.7). The narrower the margin between the two values, the more confident we can be that the relationship between the variables is statistically significant.

Box 8.7 An example of a study with confidence intervals

Mathews et al. (2008) used 95% CI to describe statistical significance in relation to the provision of personal protective equipment and safety devices to prevent blood exposure to paramedics. In the whole of the United States 96% of respondents said that safety intravenous devices were always provided (95% CI 95–97). This narrow confidence interval reassures us that we can have a high degree of confidence in the significance of this finding.

Using a quantitative research critiquing tool

Within the health service, there is a continuous drive for quality care based on the best available current evidence. Although not the only source of evidence, research material is an invaluable resource. However, not all research is good research and it is important that there are mechanisms whereby the quality of published research can be appraised. A critiquing tool utilises a framework or checklist to appraise the quality of a study. Such tools should address the following:

- the focus of the research and the research question

- the research approach

- sample selection and recruitment

- bias
- extraneous variables
- *confounding factors*
- findings – are they statistically significant? Can they be generalised to your workplace?
- congruence with findings of other studies.

Useful, tried and tested frameworks such as the Clinical Appraisal Skills Programme (CASP) have been devised and are freely available (Public Health Resource Unit 2006). This is discussed further in Chapter 5.

Conclusion

This chapter has provided an introduction to quantitative research and basic statistical concepts. Hopefully, those of you who wish to take the first steps into conducting your own research will now be more confident in posing a suitable research question and developing your hypotheses. For those of you who have no desire at present to embark on your own research project, the chapter should help you get more out of reading and appraising quantitative research papers.

The chapter has highlighted that quantitative research is not one single approach to research. Rather, it is an umbrella term that incorporates both experimental and non-experimental studies. The final choice of method should be determined by the research question. Chapter 9 will build on the material discussed in this chapter.

References

Bowling, A. (2005) Quantitative social science: the survey. In: Bowling, A. and Ebrahim, S. (eds) (2005) *Handbook of Health Research Methods: Investigation, Measurement and Analysis.* Maidenhead: Open University Press.

Bowling, A. (2009) *Research Methods in Health. Investigating Health and Health Services* (3rd edn). Trowbridge: Redwood Books.

Bryman, A. (2008) *Social Research Methods* (3rd edn). Oxford: Oxford University Press.

Chen, L. and Hsiao, A.L. (2008) Randomized trial of endotracheal tube versus laryngeal mask airway in simulated prehospital pediatric arrest. *Pediatrics* 122(2): e294–297.

Jones, A.P., Allison, K., Wright, H. and Porter, K. (2008) Use of prehospital dressings in soft tissue trauma: is there any conformity or plan? *Emergency Medical Journal* 26: 532–535.

Lerner, E.B., Fernandez, A.R. and Shah, M.N. (2009) Do EMS professionals think they should participate in disease prevention? *Prehospital Emergency Care* 13(1): 64–70.

Mathews, R., Leiss, J.K., Lyden, J.T., Sousa, S., Ratcliffe, J.M. and Jagger, J. (2008) Provision and use of personal protective equipment and safety devices in the National Study to Prevent Blood Exposure in Paramedics. *American Journal of Infection Control* 36: 743–749.

Oppenheim, A.N. (1992) *Questionnaire Design, Interviewing and Attitude Measurement* (2nd edn). London: Cassell.

Parahoo, A.K. (2006) *Nursing Research, Process and Issues* (2nd edn). London: Macmillan Press.

Polit, D. and Beck, C. (2008) *Nursing Research: Generating and Assessing Evidence for Nursing Practice* (8th edn). Philadelphia, CA: Lippincott, Williams and Wilkins.

Public Health Resource Unit (2006) *Appraisal Tools*. http://www.phru.nhs.uk/Pages/PHD/resources.htm

Rajabali, N.A., Tsuyuki, R.T., Sookram, S., Simpson, S.H. and Welsh, R.C. (2008) Evaluation of attitudes and perceptions of key clinical stakeholders regarding out-of-hospital diagnosis and treatment of ST elevation myocardial infarction patients using a region-wide survey. *Emergency Medical Journal* 26: 371–376.

Siriwardena, A.N., Iqbal, M., Banerjee, S., Spaight, A. and Stephenson, J. (2009) An evaluation of an educational intervention to reduce inappropriate cannulation and improve cannulation technique by paramedics. *Emergency Medical Journal* 26: 831–836.

Additional reading

Hek, G. and Moule, P. (2006) *Making Sense of Research. An Introduction for Health and Social Care Practitioners* (3rd edn). London: Sage.

Maltby, J., Day, L. and Williams, G. (2007) *Introduction to Statistics for Nurses*. Harlow: Pearson Education.

Roethlisberger, F.S. and Dickson, W.J. (1939) *Management and the Worker*. Boston, MA: Harvard University Press.

9 Using quantitative research methods in paramedic practice

Jayne Cutter

Learning outcomes for the chapter

By the end of this chapter the reader should be able to:

1   Differentiate between experimental and non-experimental research

2   Understand how to identify an appropriate method to address a research question

3   Understand how to select the most appropriate means of data collection for the study

4   Recognise the difference between research, clinical audit and service evaluation

Keywords

clinical audit
data collection
quantitative
research approach
service evaluation

Introduction

In the previous chapter, we established that quantitative research is used where variables can be measured and relationships between them examined objectively. Quantitative studies are concerned with empirical evidence and the findings reflect reality rather than beliefs. They are therefore suitable for situations where information can be gathered using structured methods, providing data that can be subjected to statistical analysis.

Quantitative research studies are either experimental or non-experimental in design. This chapter will explore both experimental and non-experimental designs and their suitability for different types of research question will be discussed. The advantages and disadvantages of the various methods will be considered and the credibility of the findings of studies utilising these methods will be appraised.

The critical issue in research is the awareness of the pertinence of particular methods. The most important question to be asked when deciding on a suitable research design either for a dissertation or research project is: 'What method will best answer the research question?' This alone should determine which approach is adopted, not: 'I don't like numbers so I won't do a quantitative study' or: 'I don't do touchy, feely, so qualitative research is out of the question'. Once what is to be investigated is carefully considered the appropriate design should become apparent. However, researchers are increasingly recognising that a single method approach may not always fully answer the research question. We must acknowledge that all research methods have flaws, and adopting a single method may involve exchanging deficiencies in one area for gains in another. Therefore, it may be necessary to approach the study with a range of appropriate methods to explore each individual issue to ensure the validity of the design and results. Hence combining two or more quantitative approaches, or even mixing quantitative with qualitative approaches, is gaining popularity.

Grimes and Schulz (2002) described a hierarchy of evidence of quantitative research designs largely based on the rigour of the design, the level of control the researcher has on the variables under consideration and the degree to which randomisation of the samples takes place (Box 9.1).

Box 9.1 Hierarchy of evidence (Grimes and Schulz 2002)

1 Cross-sectional study – a snapshot in time

2 Cohort study – looking forward in time

3 Case control study – thinking backwards

4 Non-randomised trial – penultimate design

5 Randomised controlled trial – gold standard

The remainder of this chapter will consider the use of these methods. You may find it beneficial to refresh your memory on the stages of quantitative research before reading this chapter (see Chapter 8, Figure 8.1).

Experimental research

Experiments are considered the pinnacle of scientific research by those who embrace the positivist paradigm who consider that 'there is a fixed orderly reality that can be objectively studied' (Polit and Beck 2008: 762). Experiments rely on the researcher manipulating the independent variable and measuring the effect on the dependent variable.

Data may be collected only once or on several occasions within the same study. Consider a study that measures the success of post-exposure prophylaxis (PEP) in preventing occupational acquisition of HIV infection following a needlestick injury. Data cannot be collected pre-needlestick injury as it would not meet the parameters set in the research question. Therefore, an after-only or post-test design would be followed where data are only collected following the injury and subsequent administration of PEP. Another popular design is the before–after or pretest–posttest design. This is the approach taken where baseline data is collected before the intervention (pretest) and then data collected following the intervention (posttest), e.g. the success of a teaching intervention in improving practice (Siriwardena et al. 2009, see Box 9.3).

Randomised controlled trials

For some researchers, the only true experiment is the randomised controlled trial (RCT). RCTs are considered the 'gold standard' study design in healthcare research for the following reasons:

- Researcher bias is minimised through randomisation of the sample into intervention and *control groups*. The intervention and control groups will contain individuals who are closely matched in terms of characteristics that may influence the findings of the study conferring a high degree of internal validity as a cause and effect relationship can be identified.

- The sample size is generally large. This increases generalisability as a large sample is more likely to be representative of the general population than a small sample. However, this does not necessarily mean that RCTs have a high degree of external validity as the participants are often selected from a narrowly defined group under certain conditions and unless the findings can be applied to a similar population within a different setting, external validity may be compromised.

- Physical behaviours or biological measurements (changes in blood pressure, response to medication) are carefully defined leaving little or no room for researcher bias to influence the findings.

- RCTs move forward in time, hence reducing bias caused by faulty memory.

- Confounding factors and variables are tightly controlled.

- The studies can be easily replicated and have a high degree of reliability.

RCTs are intended to determine the success of an intervention, e.g. the success of a drug compared to a *placebo* in treating a defined medical condition or the effect of different interventions. Participants are put into an experimental or control group randomly to prevent bias. Researchers are often unaware (or blind) to which group is receiving the intervention. This is known as a *single blind study*. On occasions both the researcher and subject are unaware of whether they are in an intervention or control group and these are known as *double blind studies*. Regardless of whether blinding is used, groups share characteristics relevant to the research study – all may have the same medical condition, share the same profession, undertake the same university course, have similar physical attributes. The only difference between groups is that the experimental group receives an intervention, e.g. a drug, teaching session, dietary supplement, while the control group either receives no intervention or a placebo. This is classified as a parallel groups or between subject design and is the commonest type of RCT.

Occasionally, there may be more than one experimental group where more than one variable is being tested, for example an experiment that examines the contribution of exercise and a calorie controlled diet on weight loss. One experimental group may be put onto a weight loss programme; the other experimental group may go onto the same weight loss programme but also be provided with an intensive exercise regimen, while the control group receives neither intervention.

Despite rigorous efforts on behalf of the researchers to recruit participants with similar characteristics, there may be times when simply being a human being may influence the outcome. Factors such as experience, prior learning, familiarity and adaptation may act as confounders and change the participants' responses over time so that the researcher can never be fully confident that it is purely the intervention that is responsible for the findings. To account for this a crossover or within subject design may be adopted in which the participants are randomly assigned to their respective groups for a period of time and then swapped so that the experimental group becomes the control group and vice versa (Box 9.2).

Box 9.2 An example of a randomised crossover study

A randomised crossover design was employed by Chen and Hsiao (2008) to investigate whether, in simulated cardiac arrest situations in children, laryngeal mask airways (LMA) resulted in shorter times to effective ventilation compared to endotracheal tubes.

Following a training session, emergency medical technicians were randomly allocated to use either the LMA or endotracheal tubes for ventilation and then the scenarios were repeated with each group using the alternate device.

Quasi-experiments

It may not always be possible to conduct an RCT because randomisation is difficult or impossible because of clinical, ethical, institutional, organisational or managerial constraints. Therefore, although the effect of interventions can still be measured, the non-intervention group is used as a comparator rather than a control. These are known as quasi-experiments as they have many of the attributes of a true experiment but as randomisation cannot be achieved, it is impossible to determine categorically that the outcome was purely the result of the intervention rather than a by-product of the differing characteristics between groups. Therefore, quasi-experiments do not have the same degree of internal validity as RCTs but nevertheless provide very interesting and pertinent data (Box 9.3).

Box 9.3 Quasi-experimental study

Siriwardena et al. (2008) performed a quasi-experimental study to evaluate the effect of an educational intervention on inappropriate cannulations and cannulation technique with paramedics from two counties in the UK.

The study followed a pretest-posttest design in that it measured cannulation technique before and after an education session provided to the intervention group only and compared the results from the intervention and comparator groups.

On occasion, a researcher may conduct a quasi-experimental study in which there is no comparator group. In this case, known as an interrupted time series experiment, a series of measurements are taken before and after an intervention on one experimental group only.

Despite the limitations of not randomising the sample, quasi-experiments perform a very useful function in healthcare research. Randomisation is often difficult or impossible in social settings. The convenience of assigning participants to groups based on workplace, place of residence etc. may outweigh the benefits of randomisation providing the researcher gives careful consideration to whether an alternative explanation can be found for the outcome. For example, in Box 9.3, one must consider whether it is likely that the characteristics of paramedics in each of the counties were likely to be sufficiently different to explain the fact that clinical practices varied between them or that the most likely explanation for the findings is that the educational intervention had a positive impact leading to improved care in the *intervention group*.

Non-experimental research

In a study where the independent variable cannot be manipulated, where an attempt to control a variable may compromise safety, experimental research cannot be undertaken and is replaced by non-experimental or observational research. For example, Leiss et al. (2009) undertook a survey to identify circumstances surrounding exposure to blood by paramedics. Variables such as the use of safety equipment and personal protective equipment and patient behaviour were identified as significant in whether exposure took place. Had the researchers wanted to know if any of these variables, e.g. wearing eye protection, was particularly likely to be significant in reducing exposures to blood, they could have considered an experiment in which one group (the experimental group) were provided with protective eyewear and another (the control group) were not allowed access to this equipment. At the end of the experiment, the number of paramedics in each group who sustained a splash of blood into their eyes could be compared to identify whether wearing eye protection significantly reduced such adverse exposures. However, despite the potential value of such an experiment, it would be entirely unethical as the efficacy of protective eyewear in reducing exposures has already been established and withholding this equipment could put paramedics at an unnecessary risk of infection.

Non-experimental research may be descriptive in that it is intended to provide information on how many of a given sample hold certain opinions. Similarly, information on how certain events and characteristics are associated with each other can be obtained from descriptive studies. Descriptive studies are often the first foray into quantitative research and can help generate hypotheses for further studies.

In *correlational research*, relationships between variables are explored without any intervention from the researcher and, despite lacking the rigour associated with experiments, can provide evidence supporting associations between changes in one variable and changes in another. However, pre-existing differences between the participants may be responsible for the findings and any apparent similarities or differences may be the result of individual factors rather than the variables under consideration. Nevertheless, as not all samples are amenable to randomisation because of ethical and other difficulties, shunning non-experimental studies because of any perceived lack of rigour would result in a lack of investigation of problems that are very significant in healthcare.

Under the umbrella of non-experimental research are various research designs and once again, it must be emphasised here that the appropriate design is the one that is best suited to answering the research question. A common distinction used to describe non-experimental research studies is whether the design is retrospective or prospective. A *retrospective study* (Chapter 8, Box 8.3) uses information from the past to explain current events. The dependent variable is identified first and the past explored to identify independent variables. One must introduce a note of caution here. Although retrospective information can be useful in explaining current phenomena, some of this information may not have been collected with research in mind and as Parahoo (2006: 193) states: 'Description of past behaviour may be highly subjective'. Nevertheless, retrospective studies have been used to explain present outcomes by considering precursors to them and can be conducted economically. See Box 9.4.

Box 9.4 An example of a retrospective (cohort) study

Boyle et al. (2008a) conducted a review of case notes of patients to identify the number and outcome of trauma patients suffering a sudden deterioration of their condition in the presence of paramedics in order to discover whether mechanism of injury is a useful predictor of deterioration and to ascertain the appropriate triage strategy for patients who deteriorate at the scene or during transport.

The study identified that very few patients suddenly deteriorated in the presence of paramedics but that those taken to a major hospital with higher trauma admissions had fewer management errors and preventable deaths. A sudden drop in blood pressure was significant in predicting deterioration.

The possibility of missing or poor quality data was identified as a limitation of the study.

Prospective studies are only concerned with exploring current phenomena by seeking information from the future. Once the research question has been identified, data collection moves forward in time. Some studies will operate a retrospective and prospective design within the same study for example, longitudinal studies in which data is collected at several points in time.

Case control studies

A case study involves detailed analysis of a single case where the term 'case' does not relate to an individual but to a location, institution, community or other group. Case studies are descriptive in nature and have a retrospective design. Case control studies (Box 9.5) compare a group of people who have an outcome of interest (case) with a group of people who do not (control) where the case is exposed to the independent variable and the control is not. Providing any characteristics that could influence the findings are very closely matched to avoid confusion, a cause and effect relationship can be established because the outcome definitely follows the exposure.

The relationship between cigarette smoking and lung cancer is well known but provides a good illustration of how case control studies can be used to establish cause and effect. Imagine if this relationship had not yet been proven, but a researcher suspected that a link existed. In order to evaluate the impact of cigarette smoking on the incidence of lung cancer, this researcher could undertake a case control study. A group of people suffering from lung cancer (the case) could be examined retrospectively to determine how many had ever smoked. A second group of people who did not have lung cancer (the control) could also be examined retrospectively to see how many of them had smoked. The two groups must be as similar as possible in every way apart from smoking. The findings could then be compared to establish whether smoking increased the likelihood of lung cancer. If more of those suffering from lung cancer had smoked in comparison to the control group, then a causal relationship between smoking and lung cancer could be established.

Box 9.5 An example of a case control study

In 2005, Chittari et al. undertook a case control study to compare prehospital thrombolytic therapy for ST elevation myocardial infarction with in-hospital thrombolytic therapy.

Patients receiving pre-hospital thrombolytic therapy (case) were compared with patients receiving the same treatment in hospital (control). Each group was matched closely in terms of age, gender and postcode.

Pre-hospital treatment resulted in much earlier delivery of treatment compared to hospital treatment.

Cohort studies

Cohort studies may be prospective or retrospective. In a prospective cohort study, the researchers begin with a presumed cause and move forward in time to identify the supposed outcome, for example whether healthcare workers who sustained a needlestick injury developed HIV infection. Prospective cohort studies are very often costly to undertake as a long study period may be required to demonstrate the effect one is investigating and a large sample size may be needed if the outcome is rare. The researcher has to be certain that all participants are initially free of the condition being studied.

Again, the example of whether cigarette smoking causes lung cancer is relevant here. A cohort study undertaken to identify whether a relationship between smoking and lung cancer exists could involve long-term follow-up of a group (or cohort) of participants, some of whom are smokers and others who are not, to determine whether any of them developed lung cancer in later life. If the incidence of lung cancer was higher in the smokers than the rest of the cohort, a link between smoking and lung cancer could be established.

Cohort studies can also employ a retrospective design (see Box 9.4) and measure exposures from the past and outcomes in the present. This approach is useful in determining how many people develop a condition rather than whether they acquired it or not, e.g. how many of a cohort of patients with diagnosed coronary heart disease died following a myocardial infarction.

Cross-sectional studies

Cross-sectional studies observe and describe what is happening within a population at a given point in time and measure both exposures and outcomes simultaneously (Box 9.6). Cross-sectional studies are retrospective and report past as well as current behaviours and attitudes. They cannot be used to establish causality as no intervention is carried out by the researcher. Consequently in cross-sectional studies, phenomena cannot be tested but can only be observed. In other words, relationships between variables are examined but the variables are not manipulated by the researcher. The exact nature of the relationship may be ambiguous as it is impossible to conclude from the results whether the exposure preceded the outcome, leading one to suspect that there may be more than one explanation for the findings.

Box 9.6 Cross-sectional study

Boyle et al. (2008b) employed a cross sectional study methodology to explore graduate paramedic students' experiences of clinical placements. A survey was conducted among a sample of which 62% were female.

Several variables were considered relating to experiences on rural and metropolitan clinical placements and whether these variables provided a positive experience clinically or educationally.

If we were interested in how many healthcare workers developed HIV infection following a needlestick injury for example, questions about HIV status and previous needlestick injuries could be posed in the same survey. If those participants who were infected reported previous needlestick injuries, it might be tempting to assume that one of these injuries was the cause of the infection. While this may be the case, cause and effect cannot be conclusively established in this example as the healthcare worker may have been HIV positive before any needlestick injuries occurred. Furthermore, they may have other risk factors such as a history of unprotected sexual intercourse or intravenous drug use which may have caused the infection rather than a needlestick injury. Cross-sectional studies therefore lack the degree of internal validity found in experimental studies.

In cross-sectional studies, data are collected within one time period, therefore they are reasonably economical to conduct and can consider several exposures and outcomes simultaneously. However, the fact that there is only one data collection period means that one cannot infer changes over time from a cross-sectional study. Data collection usually involves undertaking a survey or structured observation. The 'falseness' of completing a questionnaire or being observed may compromise ecological validity but the very nature of these structured data collection methods means that cross-sectional studies can be easily replicated by other researchers or within different populations.

Data collection in non-experimental studies

Data collection in descriptive and correlational studies may involve a number of strategies. Retrospective review of existing information including archived material, case notes and health records will provide a wealth of information useful for hypothesis formation and describing phenomena. Rigid criteria must be applied when examining such material to ensure that a systematic approach is taken. Where 'new' data is required, studies commonly employ surveys or direct observation. In the previous chapter, we considered how these can be used to effectively collect data. Despite the evident advantages, however, we have to acknowledge that there are some limitations to both surveys and observation. Next, we will consider their potential disadvantages and how we can minimise their effects.

Survey

Response rates in surveys, particularly postal and email surveys, are notoriously low although Parahoo (2006) acknowledges that it is difficult to define how many responses are acceptable. A zero response rate is theoretically possible, for example, in those in vulnerable groups, e.g. those with serious mental illness. A poor response rate means that the quality of the data may be compromised and the results may not be representative of the population being studied since the opinions of the non-responders may be vastly different from those who responded (Bryman 2008). (See Box 9.7). In addition, a low response rate can compromise the external validity of the data set.

Box 9.7 An example of a response rate in a questionnaire survey

Mackenzie et al. (2008) undertook a questionnaire survey to explore views regarding the provision of pre-hospital critical care in the UK. Thirty-two respondents took part, giving a response rate of 40%.

The authors acknowledge that the low response rate may have introduced bias as those who chose not to respond may have held very different views from those who took part.

Some respondents may be 'people pleasers' and respond to a questionnaire in the way that they think will satisfy the researcher. These responses may reflect professional norms and values, i.e. this is the way a paramedic should think/respond/act. In survey research, the researcher may introduce or perceive a degree of bias when interviewing a subject perhaps due to facial expression, tone of voice or the way in which a question or answer is phrased. The use of standardised questions reduces the risk of bias and this is further reduced when surveys are conducted in the absence of the researcher. Ambiguity may be a problem if the wording on the questionnaire is misleading and as there is no researcher present to clarify the meaning, confusion may result in inappropriate responses and poor quality data. Therefore, those embarking on a project that will collect data via survey, questionnaire design and strategies aimed at improving response rates become very important. The following should be considered (Oppenheim 1992; McColl et al. 2001; Bryman 2008; Edwards et al. 2009):

- Use financial or other incentives. These do not have to be large but may encourage participation.

- Keep the questionnaires short, balancing the need to obtain as much relevant information as possible and compiling a questionnaire which deters potential respondents from completing it because of its length.

- In postal surveys, the fact that there is no interviewer present to create a rapport with respondents means that the questionnaire itself has to keep respondents motivated rather than encouragement from a third person. Keep it snappy, relevant and interesting to the study population.

- Make letters and questionnaires personal. Using a stamp rather than having the letter commercially franked also adds a 'personal touch'.

- Contacting participants before sending questionnaires also builds a relationship and encourages participation.

- Provide clear instructions. The researcher will not be with the respondent when a postal questionnaire is completed.

- Send the questionnaire by first class post to emphasise the importance of the study.

- Follow-up contact of non-responders is useful but must be balanced against the likelihood that too much contact will antagonise those who do not want to participate.

- Non-threatening questions such as gender, age, etc. should be listed at the beginning of a questionnaire.

- A questionnaire that appears cluttered or crowded may discourage respondents; keep it simple.

- Ensure anonymity and confidentiality.

Observation

In the previous chapter, we considered how observation is a useful method for collecting data where self-reporting may be impossible or inaccurate. For example, a study designed to explore blood exposure events among paramedics could utilise a questionnaire survey to ask the participants to report on circumstances surrounding the events. This was the approach taken by Leiss et al. (2009). Individuals may however under-report the number of injuries because of recall bias, fear of censure, the social desirability response or reluctance to report on events where a failure to follow the correct procedure may have been a contributory factor. Direct observation of practices 'in the field' would eliminate erroneous reporting although this method is not without its own limitations.

Four types of observer have been described by Gold (1958) and each has its own advantages and disadvantages:

- The *complete observer*. Here the researcher acts in the capacity of complete observer by observing the participants without intervening in any way and without being noticed, or complete participant by participating in events without revealing that he/she is undertaking research. Ethical difficulties arise in that the observation must be covert. None of the participants are aware that they are being observed, and while this might yield data that accurately reflects true behaviour, this type of data collection might be interpreted as deceptive and may be fraught with ethical difficulties (see Chapter 4).

- The *observer as participant*. In this case the observer participates in the activity being observed, perhaps as a fellow healthcare worker. However, the researcher in the capacity of complete participant could be faced with ethical or moral concerns if unsafe practices are observed. Is it negligent to continue to observe without intervention if safety is compromised? This may also apply to the complete participant.

- The *participant as observer* or complete participant. When the researcher becomes a participant as observer or observer as participant, his/her presence is likely to influence the behaviour of those being studied, a phenomenon commonly known as the **Hawthorne effect** first described by Roethlisberger and Dickson (1939). It is possible, however, working on the principle that familiarity breeds acceptance, that eventually those being studied become accustomed to the presence of the researcher and begin to behave naturally because it is difficult to behave in an artificial manner for too long.

When observation is employed the issue of observer bias becomes a potential threat. It is difficult for a researcher to remove themselves completely from the situation being observed and emotions, memories, experiences and prejudices may all influence the way in which the situation is perceived. For those who are very familiar with the situation being observed, it is possible that they may see what they expect to see rather than what is actually happening.

Clinical audit and service evaluations

Audit is not research however; research and audit share many of the same aspirations and, on occasion, employ the same methodology. Both adopt a rigorous and systematic approach towards addressing a problem or situation but while healthcare research endeavours to find new knowledge with the intention of improving care, audit is concerned with improving services by comparing practices against a pre-existing standard and as such reviews the quality of current interventions rather than seeking to find new ones. These differences notwithstanding, audit provides data that are applicable to practical healthcare situations with the intention of improving practice.

Service evaluations aim to improve the service provided to service users based on an evaluation of current practice by soliciting opinion from service users or service providers and once again may employ the same data collection or data analysis methods as research.

The overlap in methods between research, audit and service evaluation can sometimes be confusing. To help you determine if your planned work is research, audit or service evaluation, the characteristics of each have been listed in Figure 9.1 and the similarities and differences between them are identified.

Conclusion

In this chapter we have considered how various approaches may be taken to quantitative data collection according to the nature of the problem one wants to investigate. The key message here is that the study design must be appropriate to the question. However, occasionally, there are factors such as accessibility of the sample and ethical considerations that may compromise the researcher's ability to adopt their preferred method, e.g. being unable to randomise a sample and having to abandon a proposed RCT in favour of a quasi-experimental study, but that this does not necessarily have a significant adverse effect on the quality and applicability of the findings.

Quantitative research has an important place in contributing to knowledge in healthcare. It has provided a pool of evidence on which paramedic science practitioners can base and improve their practice as illustrated by the examples in Boxes 9.2–9.7.

Characteristic	Research	Clinical audit	Service evaluation
Intended outcome is improved knowledge	Yes	No	No
Intended outcome is improved quality of practice	Indirectly	Yes	Yes
Approval from a Research Ethics Committee required	Yes	Not usually	No
May be based on a hypothesis	Yes	No	No
Randomisation of sample	In RCT, otherwise no	No	No
Involves experiments on human subjects	Sometimes	No	No
May be invasive	Sometimes	No	No
May test a new practice, intervention, therapy or drug	Yes	No	No
May involve collecting data from medical records	Yes	Yes	No
May employ interviews or questionnaires for data collection	Yes	Yes	Yes
May involve changes to normal clinical management	Yes	No	No
Involves comparison of practice against current standards	No	Yes	No
Results may change practice if new interventions, tests or therapies are shown to be effective	Yes	No	No
May employ statistical analysis	Yes	Yes	Yes
Findings are transferrable to other clinical settings	Yes	No	No

Figure 9.1 Characteristics of research, clinical audit and service evaluation

References

Boyle, M.J., Smith, E.C. and Archer, F. (2008a) A review of patients who suddenly deteriorate in the presence of paramedics. *BMC Emergency Medicine* 8: 9. Available at http://www.biomedcentral.com/1471-227X-8-9 [accessed 9 July 2010]

Boyle, M.J., Williams, B., Cooper, J., Adams, B. and Alford, K. (2008b) Ambulance clinical placements – a pilot study of students' experience. *BMC Medical Education*. 8: 19. Available at http://www.biomedcentral.com/1472-6920/8/19 [accessed 9 July 2010]

Bryman, A. (2008) *Social Research Methods* (3rd edn). Oxford: Oxford University Press.

Chen, L. and Hsiao, A.L. (2008) Randomized trial of endotracheal tube versus laryngeal mask airway in simulated prehospital pediatric arrest. *Pediatrics* 122(2): e294–297.

Chittari, M.S.V.M., Ahmad, I., Chambers, B., Knight, F., Scriven, A. and Pitcher, D. (2005) Retrospective observational case-control study comparing prehospital thrombolytic therapy for ST-elevation myocardial infarction with in-hospital thrombolytic therapy for patients from same area. *Emergency Medical Journal* 22: 582–585.

Edwards, P.J., Roberts, I. and Clarke, M.J. (2009) Methods to increase response to postal and electronic questionnaires. *Cochrane Database Systematic Review*. Jul 8;(3): MR000008. Available at http://www.ncbi.nlm.nih.gov/pubmed/19588449 [accessed 9 July 2010]

Gold, R. (1958) Roles in sociographic field investigation. *Social Forces* 36: 217–223.

Grimes, D.A. and Schulz, K.F. (2002) An overview of clinical research: the lay of the land. *Lancet* 359: 57–61.

Leiss, J.K., Sousa, S. and Boal, W.L. (2009) Circumstances surrounding occupational blood exposure events in the national study to prevent blood exposure in paramedics. *Industrial Health* 27: 139–44.

McColl, E., Jacoby, A., Thomas, L. et al. (2001) Design and use of questionnaires: a review of best practice applicable to surveys of health service staff and patients. *Health Technology Assessment* 5(31): 1–256.

Mackenzie, R., Steel, A., French, J. et al. (2008) Views regarding the provision of prehospital critical care in the UK. *Emergency Medical Journal* 26: 365–370.

Oppenheim, A.N. (1992) *Questionnaire Design, Interviewing and Attitude Measurement* (2nd edn). London: Cassell.

Parahoo, A.K. (2006) *Nursing Research, Process and Issues* (2nd edn). London: Macmillan Press.

Polit, D. and Beck, C. (2008) *Nursing Research: Generating and Assessing Evidence for Nursing Practice* (8th edn). Philadelphia, CA: Lippincott, Williams and Wilkins.

Roethlisberger, F.S. and Dickson, W.J. (1939) *Management and the Worker*. Boston, MA: Harvard University Press.

Siriwardena, A.N., Iqbal, M., Banerjee, S., Spaight, A. and Stephenson, J. (2009) An evaluation of an educational intervention to reduce inappropriate cannulation and improve cannulation technique by paramedics. *Emergency Medical Journal* 26: 831–836.

Recommended reading

Bowling, A. (2009) *Research Methods in Health: Investigating Health and Health Services* (3rd edn). Trowbridge: Open University Press.

Bowling, A. and Ebrahim, S. (eds) (2005) *Handbook of Health Research Methods: Investigation, Measurement and Analysis*. Maidenhead: Open University Press.

Denscombe, M. (2003) *The Good Research Guide for Small Scale Social Projects* (2nd edn). Buckingham: Open University Press.

Hek, G. and Moule, P. (2006) *Making Sense of Research: An Introduction for Health and Social Care Practitioners* (3rd edn). London: Sage.

Liamputtong, P. (ed.) (2010) *Research Methods in Health. Foundations for Evidence Based Practice*. Melbourne: Oxford University Press.

Maltby, J., Day, L. and Williams, G. (2007) *Introduction to Statistics for Nurses*. Harlow: Pearson Education.

National Institute for Health and Clinical Excellence (NICE) (2002) *Principles for Best Practice in Clinical Audit, National Institute for Clinical Excellence*. Available at: http://www.nice.org.uk/pdf/BestPracticeClinicalAudit.pdf

10 Researching paramedic clinical practice: a practical guide

Malcolm Woollard and Julia Williams

Learning outcomes for the chapter
By the end of this chapter the reader should be able to:

1 Understand the purpose of clinical research

2 Recognise potential funding sources for pre-hospital research

3 Outline the differences between peer-reviewed and professional journals

4 Understand some of the challenges encountered when disseminating research through a variety of methods including journal publication and conference presentations

Keywords
clinical practice
funding
publishing
research projects

Introduction

It seems reasonable to suggest that paramedics, as clinicians, are likely to be most interested in research that changes their clinical practice for the better. The body of knowledge that underpins pre-hospital care is generalist, extending across a broad range of disciplines, but is applied in the highly specialised and challenging out-of-hospital setting. The paramedic profession is also relatively new, certainly in comparison to medicine and nursing, and its members have only comparatively recently started to undertake academic education. It is not surprising, therefore, that the amount of research undertaken around pre-hospital care is limited and rarely of the most robust quality.

At the core of Department of Health policy is that clinical practice should be evidence based. The predominant role of clinical research is therefore to:

- eliminate treatments where risk outweighs benefit – and which are therefore harmful

- eliminate treatments which have no benefit – and which are therefore ineffective (since continuing to fund these represents an *opportunity cost* – the monies used cannot be spent instead on an effective treatment)

- increase the number of treatments with clear evidence of benefits outweighing risks – and which therefore do good

- reduce the number of treatments for which efficacy is not proven – and where the ratio of benefit to risk is unknown.

Not all clinical interventions can or should be researched: for example, there has never been a randomised controlled trial of pre-hospital defibrillation in UK pre-hospital care. The benefits are clear from observed practice and it would therefore be unethical to randomise half of all patients in ventricular fibrillation to a control group. On the other hand, observation alone is rarely sufficient to 'prove' that treatment is effective. Tepid sponging has been recommended for the treatment of febrile convulsions, and in particular to prevent second fits, for many years. Most clinicians who have used this intervention would argue that they know it is effective because whenever they have implemented it the child being treated has not fitted again. But this is in fact *association* being misinterpreted as *causation*. The definition of a febrile convulsion is a single fit in a 24-hour period associated with a rapid rise in temperature. By definition a child with a febrile convulsion will only fit once, but observation by a clinician unaware of this fact may lead them to conclude that *any* treatment they had given was the reason the child did not fit again. In this case only a randomised controlled study with half of the febrile children randomly assigned to tepid sponging and the other half to no tepid sponging would identify that the recommended treatment had no effect.

Due to their desire to improve patient outcome, paramedics are typically very enthusiastic about new equipment purporting to improve patient outcome, and there have been many instances in the past of considerable investment being made in the absence of robust evidence of benefit. A recent example of this is the use of mechanical chest compression devices. Intuitively these do seem to have the potential to improve out-of-hospital cardiac arrest survival. The quality of manual chest compressions can be very poor, even when provided by health professionals, the quality starts to deteriorate within one minute, and there are frequent long gaps in compressions whilst other procedures are performed and clinicians are distracted (Hightower et al. 1995). A mechanical device should eliminate these problems: but this cannot be interpreted as meaning that more patients will survive to discharge (Perkins et al. 2010). Does this matter if it makes cardio-pulmonary resuscitation easier? Of course – a mechanical device might cause injury and therefore worsen outcome. Even if it makes no difference, purchasing ineffective equipment results in an *opportunity cost* – simply meaning that the money spent on ineffective devices is no longer available to spend on equipment of proven efficacy. Other issues worthy of exploration in relation to mechanical chest compression could include, for example, paramedics' experiences of using this equipment and identification of factors that influence their decision to use this mechanical device.

In summary, paramedics have the opportunity to undertake research to improve their practice and patient care by:

- investigating treatments that are currently in use but for which there is no robust evidence of benefit

- investigating new ways of using existing equipment or drugs in the pre-hospital setting

- investigating equipment or drugs that are used in other settings (such as in hospital practice) before they are widely adopted in pre-hospital care

- developing and evaluating new equipment for use in the pre-hospital setting

- exploring people's experiences, thinking and behaviours in order to understand a variety of phenomena in the pre-hospital setting

- examining factors which influence paramedics' clinical decision making

- exploring existing culture(s) in pre-hospital care to better understand the complexities of the unscheduled urgent care environment.

Identifying research questions from practice

All good clinicians are reflective – simply meaning that after every patient contact they ask themselves if the care provided could have been improved (Blaber 2008). Often the answer will be 'no', sometimes a learning need will be identified, and sometimes a research opportunity will come to mind. For example, a paramedic experiences difficulty in gaining intra-osseous access to administer benzylpenicillin to a child who has suspected meningococcal septicaemia. Although there are a number of devices designed to place a cannula in bone to facilitate drug administration, a literature search may not find any research that compares their efficacy and ease of use. A need for research to address a problem from clinical practice has been identified.

Reading other clinicians' published research also helps to generate ideas, since most papers include a statement starting 'Further research is required to ...' in their Conclusions section. Another option is to include the public, patients and/or carers in the development of research questions at the very beginning. Service users bring a unique perspective to pre-hospital research as frequently they have been recipients of care and management by paramedics in a pre-hospital setting. Increasingly funding bodies and ethics committees expect to see early engagement of patients and the public in research projects. Working collaboratively with patients and lay representatives throughout the research process can be an extremely rewarding experience and it is important that their contributions are valued as much as those from healthcare professionals. Researchers must really embrace the challenges of partnership working and must not include lay representatives just because it looks good! Organisations such as INVOLVE promote public involvement in NHS, public health and social care research and provides useful resources and clear guidelines for good practice to help researchers develop effective methods of incorporating public opinion into research developments. See INVOLVE's website at www.invo.org.uk.

Undertaking small-scale research projects

Educational research

If you are undertaking a paramedic degree or a higher degree you may be required to undertake a research project as part of your assessment. This small-scale research is unlikely to attract funding but can still be a useful contribution to paramedic practice development. The largest cost in any study relates to staff time be it funded or non-funded.

Funding

Finding funding for any form of research is highly competitive, and few organisations focus their grants on pre-hospital care. However, some organisations with an appropriate interest are shown in Table 10.1.

Table 10.1 Potential funders of pre-hospital research

Organisation	Area of interest	Website
Resuscitation Council (UK)	Resuscitation – training, equipment, drugs, manual interventions	http://www.resus.org.uk/pages/resacts.htm
The Laerdal Foundation for Acute Medicine	Resuscitation – training, equipment, drugs, manual interventions	http://www.laerdalfoundation.org/strategi.html
Higher Education Academy	Education-related topics	http://www.health.heacademy.ac.uk/projects/miniprojects
Diabetes UK	Diabetes	http://www.diabetes.org.uk/Research/For-researchers/
The Stroke Association	Stroke/TIA	http://www.stroke.org.uk/research/apply_for_funding/

An excellent source of funding ideas is RDFunding (www.rdfunding.org.uk), part of the RDInfo web pages of the National Institute for Health Research (NIHR). As well as browsing opportunities available currently, you can also sign up for funding alerts.

Many researchers start off their research career by working in a larger team led by a senior researcher where they learn their craft and develop their publishing profile so that in time novice researchers want to work with them.

Dissemination

No research project has been completed until its findings have been disseminated: indeed it is unethical not to do so as this would represent wasted resources and a pointless exposure of research participants to risk (however small). Findings should always be distributed to study participants, with sufficient detail and couched in appropriate language to make them accessible to the intended audience. For example, it would not be helpful to copy a scientific paper to the majority of patients, although this might be appropriate for clinicians.

Writing for publication

As a clinician, there are two types of journal that you can aim to publish in: peer-reviewed and professional (non-peer-reviewed). The editor of the latter will typically accept any well-written article that will be of interest to their readers. The former has a multi-layered process for reviewing papers to quality-assure the paper. Initially a paper will be reviewed by the editor to ensure that it might be of interest to their journal's audience and is in compliance with any pre-existing editorial policies. Many papers may be rejected outright at this stage. It is important to always consider that your paper may be good but that it just was not what they were looking for at that time. Those papers that are sent on for peer-review may be rejected following this process or accepted for publication, albeit usually following a request for revisions to the original manuscript.

Although there is some overlap between the two types of journal, as a general rule writers are encouraged to publish their research in the highest 'quality' peer-reviewed journal with an audience likely to be interested in the subject you have investigated. A journal's quality or status is measured by its 'impact factor', which is derived from the number of times papers published in a journal are cited (referenced) in subsequent peer-reviewed articles. The specialist *Emergency Medicine Journal* had an impact factor of 1.477 in 2009, whereas the *BMJ* with its very broad audience had an impact factor of 13.66. However, the readership of professional journals may be far higher than that of a very academic journal and so reach a wider audience.

Another key difference between professional and peer-reviewed journals is 'indexing'. Only papers published in peer-reviewed journals are listed in databases such as Medline and CINAHL, although it is also true that not all peer-reviewed journals are indexed until they are established and meet certain criteria. The important point is that your paper will not be found via an electronic search of a clinical database unless it has been published in an indexed journal. It should also be remembered that journals might appear in one index and not another.

Structure of papers

The first stage in writing for any journal is to select the journal and read the instructions for authors usually found on the journal's website or in the journal itself. These instructions will specify how papers should be formatted with respect to headings, fonts, tables, figures and references, and will also give the maximum permitted word length and instructions on how to submit your article (almost always via an online system). Failing to follow these instructions (which vary significantly from journal to journal) is likely to result in your paper being returned without review. It is also very helpful to read recent copies of the journal to get a feel for its style, and journals encourage potential contributors to contact the editor to discuss their ideas.

Publications in peer-reviewed journals are usually required to be in IMRaD format (Introduction, Methods, Results and Discussion). A typical structure required for a paper reporting is as follows:

- Title page, to include
  - the title, which should be as short as possible but should: state what the paper is about; include the design of the study undertaken
  - the names and main organisational affiliations of all authors (authors' titles, job roles and qualifications may be asked for)
  - the name, address, email and phone number of the corresponding author (not necessarily the first author in sequence, but the person who will deal with all correspondence from the journal and its readers)
  - the word count (usually excluding the abstract, tables and references)
  - key terms (usually up to five words or short phrases which describe what your paper is about) – ideally MeSH terms to ensure your paper is cited accurately in databases such as Medline (see http://www.ncbi.nlm.nih.gov/mesh for a database of MeSH terms)
- Abstract (usually no more than 250–300 words). If your paper is describing the results of research, this should be structured – for example
  - aim – describing what question your research set out to answer
  - methods – succinctly describing how you carried out your research and including population (what group you recruited from, e.g. 'adult patients with asthma'); research design (e.g. 'randomised controlled trial'; 'ethnography' etc.), intervention; and data collection methods e.g. interviews, diaries, questionnaire
  - results/findings – including descriptive (e.g. 1/10 patients. . .) and inferential statistics (p values and confidence intervals) for quantitative research; and key codes and/or categories and/or themes for qualitative research
  - conclusions – a summary of the main findings and, where appropriate, their implications for practice.

Check carefully the authors' guidance; for peer-reviewed journals the reviewers read the papers 'blind'. This means that your name and other details are placed in a separate file that does not go to the reviewer.

- Introduction – see the usual length in the journal usually no longer than one to two sides of double-spaced A4 and will include:
  - a brief critical summary of what was known about the topic that has been researched (referencing only *key* papers – this is not a literature review)
  - a justification for the current study having been carried out: the *size* of the problem (e.g. 'cardiac arrest occurs in 1 in 115,000 people each year'); the

severity of the problem (e.g. 'only 5% of victims of out-of-hospital cardiac arrest survive to discharge')

o end the introduction with a one sentence statement of the aim of your research

- Methods – provides sufficient detail to allow another researcher to replicate your study. Sub-headings are useful but not essential. References are only given for the data the sample size calculation is based on and unusual methods
  o Design (e.g. 'randomised controlled trial'; mixed methods)
    - Describe how participants were randomised to treatments if appropriate
    - Describe, if appropriate, how participants, researchers, and statisticians were blinded to treatment allocations (or if not, why not)
    - Describe how the different components of a mixed methods study fit together to enhance understanding and/ôr explanation
    - Identify the different methods of data collection used in the study e.g. observation; questionnaire; interview; diaries and so on
  o Participants: *who* (e.g. 'adult patients with asthma attended by an emergency ambulance') and *where* (e.g. 'large UK ambulance service'); *inclusion* and *exclusion* criteria
  o Interventions – what *exactly* was done in intervention and control groups
  o Outcomes: *primary* (main outcome – e.g. 'survival to hospital discharge') and *secondary* (everything else – e.g. 'survival at 12 months, neurological status, length of hospital stay')
  o Ethics approval and consent
    - The name of the ethics committee approving the study (or state why no ethics approval was necessary)
    - Describe how informed consent was obtained
  o For quantitative research, include a sample size (power) calculation
  o For quantitative research describe what statistical tests were used for which outcome variables
  o For qualitative research identify which approach has guided your analysis (e.g. thematic analysis; constant comparison analysis; discourse analysis) and how. Maintain transparency in relation to how the data was deconstructed and coded/categorised/unitised.
  o For qualitative research outline what activities have been undertaken to facilitate data processing such as identification of computer assisted qualitative data analysis software, or description of systems of manual coding/categorisation

- Results/findings
  o Number of participants and demographics (age, gender, co-morbidity, etc. – if more than one group, these factors should be compared to identify heterogeneity [differences])
  o Recruitment – report protocol violations (e.g. recruitment of a participant not meeting the inclusion criteria); treatment allocation out of the randomisation sequence (i.e. patient allocated to treatment B but given treatment A); missing data. All patients and all data MUST be accounted for (Figure 10.1: Example of a CONSORT flowchart)

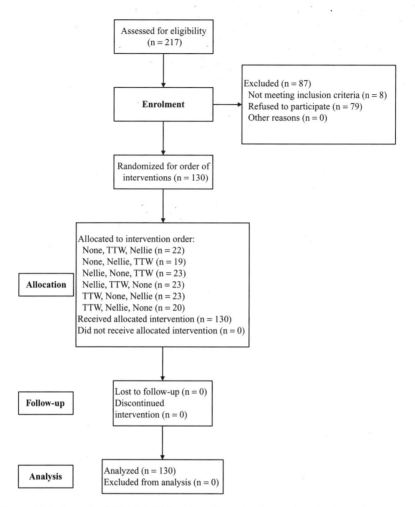

Figure 10.1 Example of CONSORT flowchart (from: Rawlins, L., Woollard, M., Williams, J. and Hallam, P. (2009) Effect of listening to Nellie the Elephant during CPR training on performance of chest compressions by lay people: randomised crossover trial. *BMJ* 339: b4707)

- ○ Outcome data
  - ▪ For quantitative data use tables comparing groups: do not duplicate data in text, but do interpret and summarise
  - ▪ Report point estimates and spread of data
    - • for parametric (normally distributed) data give means, 95% confidence intervals, and p values
    - • for non-parametric data report medians or modes and inter-quartile ranges and ranges plus p values

- In qualitative research it is important to indicate clearly when the text includes a direct citation from a primary source such as verbatim narrative from participants; or extracts from participants' diaries; researcher's field notes etc. This is frequently achieved by changing the font or the formatting of the relevant section of text using techniques such as indenting.
  - Qualitative research can seem to be more accessible and meaningful to the reader through the logical combination of the results and discussion sections as this, at the very least, avoids unnecessary repetition of data. Some journals are more empathetic to this approach than others.
  - Explicit inclusion of raw data is useful not only to illustrate discussion points but also to support the researcher's interpretation of the data and increase its credibility.

- Qualitative researchers must clearly document processes and influences involved in moving from the collection of the raw data through to the interpretation of the data and the subsequent reconstruction and recontextualisation of the data.

- Discussion
  - Start with a *brief* summary (two or three sentences) of your main findings
  - Compare and contrast your findings with a critical review of previous similar research (but do NOT attempt an exhaustive review)
    - Discuss the possible causes of any disparities
  - Discuss any limitations
    - Discuss how these affect the interpretation of your results or findings
  - End with a conclusion
    - Identify any areas for further research (do not put this last as it weakens the impact of your own research findings)
    - State what your research has added to the body of knowledge
    - State any recommendations for practice

- Acknowledge all contributors, e.g. data collectors, participants, colleagues, advisors.

- Funding – acknowledge sources of funding, stating the role of sponsors in the study (if none, say so).

- Conflict of interests
  - *Always* declare (even if only potential) or state *none* exists when professional judgement concerning a primary interest (e.g. patients' welfare or the validity of research) may be influenced by a secondary interest (such as financial gain or personal rivalry)
  - It may arise for the authors of an article when they have a financial interest that may influence their interpretation of their results or those of others
  - Not inherently unethical but should be acknowledged and openly stated

- References
  - Carefully follow the journal's style for numbering (Vancouver style) or author name and date (Harvard) in the text and in the reference list

○ Make sure these are accurate in the text and on the reference list – this is your responsibility and not the journal's.

Authorship

The vexed issue of who should be named as an author of a paper, and what order authors' names should appear in, has ruined many an academic relationship. Fortunately there is guidance on this which is followed by most journal editors (see International Committee of Medical Journal Editors. *Uniform Requirements for Manuscripts Submitted to Biomedical Journals: Writing and Editing for Biomedical Publication*, Updated October 2004 (online). Available at: http://www.icmje.org/#author). In order to qualify as an author each person must have contributed to *all three* of the following:

- conception and design or acquisition of data, or analysis and interpretation of data, *and*
- drafting the article or revising it critically for important intellectual content, *and*
- final approval of the version to be published.

Anyone not meeting these criteria should be named as a contributor in the 'Acknowledgments' section, but note that all persons who do meet these criteria MUST appear as authors unless they choose not to do so.

Writing style

- Always keep your intended audience in mind, but use simple English, avoiding jargon and pomposity.
- Spell out abbreviations in full the first time you use them.
- Pay careful attention to spelling and grammar and use short sentences.
- If you are submitting a *quant*itative paper write it in the third person (e.g. 'It could be argued that' not 'I think'). Often, however, *qual*itative research findings are presented in the first person (e.g. 'It was clear from the outset of data collection that my role would be complex'). (As always, check the guidelines of the relevant journal.)
- Remember to check your use of tenses and be sure you are consistent throughout your paper.
- Most journals require measurements to be presented in SI units.
- For proportions, give numbers first, then percentages (e.g. 10/100 [10%]).
- Check the reference numbers in your text relate to the correct reference in the list at the end, and do the same for tables and figures.
- Do not make unsupported statements such as 'all paramedics agree...'.
- Do not misuse capitals.

- Do use 'they' instead of 'he' or 'she'.

- Most of all follow the journal's instructions on style – reading papers they have previously published can provide a good reference point.

Peer-review process

Peer-reviewers are rarely trained for their role and usually are not required to have any particular qualifications. Rather they are drawn from clinicians with an interest in the journal's subject, who have been published in the journal, and who volunteer for the task. The journal's website will have information on the criteria that reviewers adhere to when considering a paper and it is helpful to be familiar with this (see Box 10.1). However, the quality of peer-reviewers' feedback can

Box 10.1 How to upset peer-reviewers

- Do not follow the instructions for authors

- Do not use spell check

- Do not explain abbreviations

- Do exceed the word count

- Do contact them directly

- Do *completely* disregard their comments

- Do be rude in your response to their comments

vary considerably, but the editor will have the ultimate responsibility of deciding whether to accept your paper and should manage any poor peer-reviewers. A good reviewer should consider the following issues:

- Is the paper important?

- Does the paper read well and make sense?

- Originality – does the work add enough to what is already in the published literature? If so, what does it add?

- Does this work matter to the intended audience (e.g. clinicians, patients, teachers or policymakers)? Is the journal in question the right place for it?

- Is the research question clearly defined and appropriately answered?

- Is the overall design of study appropriate?

- Are the participants studied adequately described and their conditions defined?

- Are the methods clearly described?

- Was the design ethical?

- Have issues of rigour been addressed within the study?

- Do the results/findings answer the research question? Are they credible and well presented?

- Were the interpretation and conclusions warranted by and sufficiently derived from/focussed on the data? Is there a clear message?

- Are the references up to date and relevant without any glaring omissions?

- Does the abstract or summary accurately reflect what the paper says?

When you receive peer-reviewers' comments on your paper, read them *carefully* and:

- Ask yourself:
  - Do the reviewers have a point?
  - How can you improve your paper based on their comments?
  - Are the reviewers wrong?
    - You do not have to make all the changes they suggest.
    - You will need to justify why if choosing not to do so.

- Always thank the peer-reviewers in the 'Acknowledgements' section

- *Never* contact the peer-reviewers directly.

- Contact the Editor for advice/clarification if necessary.

- If asked to revise and re-submit do so promptly
  - Provide a point-by-point response to all reviewers' comments.
  - Upload a revised copy of your manuscript showing 'tracked changes'.

- The Editor's decision is final (although you can sometimes lodge a rebuttal).

If you successfully negotiate all the hurdles and your paper is accepted, sometime later (it can be several months), you will receive a set of proofs which you are usually required to respond to within 48 hours of their being sent to you. You will find that a professional copyeditor will have edited your manuscript to comply with the style requirements of the journal, so check *very* carefully

- for accuracy

- verifying the reference order

- double-checking figures and tables

- making only minor changes to correct typographical errors (too late to amend your results/findings!).

You will also be asked to respond to any queries the technical editor has – such as errors in references or the failure to spell out abbreviations the first time they appear.

Publication ethics

Publication ethics in medical journals is regulated by the Committee on Publication Ethics (COPE) (see http://publicationethics.org/). This organisation helps to set generic standards and also acts as a forum for communication between journals with different publishers – ensuring that if an author behaves in a particularly unethical manner their details will be widely distributed.

The following are things to avoid when publishing in peer-reviewed journals:

- redundant publication
- more than 10% of the paper previously published elsewhere
- duplicate publication – not permitted, viewed very gravely
- simultaneous submission – not permitted, viewed very gravely
- plagiarism – always reference the work of others and yourself.

Journal editors have a number of sanctions at their disposal for the management of publication misconduct. In cases where this is suspected, editors can:

- contact authors for an explanation
  - request raw data from the study
  - request copies of study correspondence
- contact employers
- contact ethics committees
- contact other journal(s) and/or COPE
- reject the paper without regard to reviews (or un-reviewed)
- refuse to consider papers by any of the authors for a period of time or permanently
- publish a statement in the journal retracting the article, and giving the reasons why.

At worst employers may consider serious misconduct as grounds for dismissal: a professional's registrant body (e.g. the HPC) may decide to investigate and impose sanctions, including striking from the register; and a university may decide to withdraw degrees. *Always* act ethically, and if in doubt, write to the editor for advice.

Authors writing about pre-hospital research may quite reasonably be concerned that a paper they publish in a peer-reviewed journal will not be seen by the majority of paramedics. In this case, after publication, the author can contact the editor to seek permission for the paper to be replicated in a professional journal. If permission is granted the paper normally needs to be published in exactly the same format in which it originally appeared and with a full reference to the peer-reviewed journal. Clearly this will need to be agreed with the editor of the professional journal.

Presentations

An excellent means of disseminating research findings is through conference presentations. They will also advertise for abstracts to be submitted which will then be peer-reviewed and the best selected for presentation. Two options are usually offered – oral and poster presentations. As with journals, authors should carefully follow the instructions for abstract format and content provided by the conference organisers. Whether or not your paper is ultimately selected for presentation you will often be provided with feedback from the peer-reviewers – this should be taken into account in preparing your presentation if appropriate, or in preparing future abstracts for submission to other conferences. If the abstract is accepted you will be expected to attend the conference.

Oral presentations

Presenters frequently use PowerPoint to help guide the audience through the presentation. Never underestimate the importance of preparation for an oral presentation.

1 avoid trying to include too much information:
   - five or six bullet points per slide
     (i) do not write in whole sentences
   - no more than one slide per minute available
   - allow two or three minutes for questions at the end

2 Avoid over-use of animations, varying fonts and colours as this distracts from your message and makes slides difficult to read:
   - be particularly cautious about using video and audio clips, as these often fail to work 'on the day' – only do so if absolutely necessary to your point
   - make sure the combination of font and background colours is readable from a distance (always review your slides before the conference!)

3 Try not to script your presentation – use the bullet points on the slides as an aide memoire to prompt you instead and engage with the audience using eye contact.

4 Structure your presentation in the same way as you did your abstract: indeed you may wish to start by cutting and pasting your abstract onto slides and editing them into bullet points:
   - the key parts will be Aims, Methods, Results/Findings, Conclusion
     (i) don't try to report your literature review or discussion in any detail
     (ii) the methods and results/findings should take up most of the paper
     (iii) remember to include implications for practice in your conclusions

5 Put your contact details on the last slide.

6 Make a point of introducing yourself to the person who is chairing your session, and ask them how they plan to manage the session (e.g. questions from the

audience after each presentation, or questions only after all presentations in the session have been made).

7 Be yourself – do not try to act a part.

8 Time will pass really quickly, and a good conference chair will keep you to your allotted slot. Planning the time that your presentation will take will pay dividends:
   • if you plan ahead you can ask a friend in the audience or the session chair to give you a warning when a certain amount of time remains so that you can ensure you get all of your key points across
   • when the chair tells you to stop, do so

9 When responding to questions:
   • try not to be defensive if someone questions your work – think about what has been said and be open-minded
   • the questioner may have misunderstood a key element of your presentation and argument
   • if you do not know the answer, say so
   • if you do not understand the question, ask for it to be rephrased
   • remember that the audience may not have heard the question, so paraphrase it before giving your answer.

Poster presentations

Designing a good poster is a talent: it is important to remember that it is an entirely visual medium. Unless you are naturally creative the temptation is to cram as many words into the available space as possible, either replicating your abstract in its entirety or the bulk of an associated paper. Instead it is better to:

1 Follow the instructions for authors carefully, particularly with respect to:
   (a) size
   (b) orientation (i.e. landscape or portrait)

2 Divide your paper into sections – Aim, Methods, Results/Findings, Conclusions:
   (a) use the minimum number of bullet points necessary to provide only the key information
   (b) avoid whole sentences if at all possible

3 Ensure your poster's title, and authors' names and affiliations stand out clearly:
   (a) consider using organisations' logos (with permission)
   (b) do not forget to thank contributors and participants (they might be attending the conference)

4 Minimise the number of different colours and fonts used:
   (a) ensure that your text is legible throughout the poster, particularly if you use a picture as background
   (b) think about the size of fonts required for the poster to be readable from a distance

5 Use pictures to illustrate the theme of your poster;
    (a) use graphs instead of tables of results
    (b) use dramatic images to draw people in to read the text

6 Always take adhesive back Velcro with you

7 If at all possible, have your poster professionally printed;
    (a) find out in advance in what format they would like the file from which they will print
    (b) consider laminating your poster for extra protection and select a matt finish to reduce glare

8 Prepare a handout to go with your poster and leave copies attached to your poster display board.

9 Use a poster tube for transportation.

In most conferences authors will be expected to stand with their poster at pre-determined times to answer questions from attendees.

Raising awareness in your professional peer-group

Apart from journal publications and presentations there are a number of methods with which to get your message out to your target audience. For example, you can send a copy of your paper/report to:

- The College of Paramedics

- The Joint Royal Colleges Ambulance Liaison Committee Guidelines Group

- The National Ambulance Services Directors of Clinical Care Committee

- The Resuscitation Council (UK)

- Special patient interest groups

Most journals will also allow you to post the abstract from your published paper on your own and/or your employing organisation's website.

Conclusion

In this chapter, the purpose of clinical research for paramedics is outlined. You have been introduced to some funding bodies that may financially support your clinical research. The main approaches to disseminating your research are covered with guidance as to how to write effective papers for publication and some useful tips for producing good oral and poster presentations for conferences. Some of the differences between peer-reviewed and professional journals are discussed but you need to decide which publication will provide the most suitable vehicle for you to get the results/findings of your study out in to the public domain.

References and further reading

Albert, T. (2000) *A–Z of Medical Writing*. London: Wiley-Blackwell.

Albert, T. (2008) *Write Effectively: A Quick Course for Busy Health Workers*. Oxford: Radcliffe Publishing.

Blaber, A.Y. (2008) Reflective practice in relation to pre-hospital care. In: Blaber, A.Y. (ed.) *Foundations for Paramedic Practice: A Theoretical Perspective*. Maidenhead: McGraw-Hill/Open University Press.

Crombie, I. (1996) *The Pocket Guide to Critical Appraisal*. London: Wiley-Blackwell.

Greenhalgh, T. (2010) *How to Read a Paper: The Basics of Evidence-Based Medicine* (4th edn). London: Wiley-Blackwell.

Hall, G.M. (2003) *How to Write a Paper* (3rd edn). London: Wiley-Blackwell.

Hall, G.M. (2006) *How to Present at Meetings* (2nd edn). London: Wiley-Blackwell.

Hanley, B., Bradburn, J., Barnes, M., et al. (2004) *Involving the Public in NHS, Public Health, and Social Care Research: Briefing Notes for Researchers* (2nd edn). Eastleigh: INVOLVE.

Hightower, D., Thomas, S.H., Keith Stone, C., Dunn, K. and March, J.A. (1995) Decay in quality of closed-chest compressions over time. *Annals of Emergency Medicine* 26(3): 300–303.

Miller, J.E. (2007) Preparing and presenting effective research posters. *Health Service Research* 42(1): 311–328.

Perkins, G.D., Brace, S.J. and Gates, S. (2010) Mechanical chest-compression devices: current and future roles. *Current Opinion in Critical Care* 16(3): 203–210.

Wager, E., Godlee, F. and Jefferson, T. (2002) *How to Survive Peer Review*. London: Wiley-Blackwell.

The future for paramedic research

Pauline Griffiths and Gail P. Mooney

Learning outcomes for the chapter
By the end of this chapter the reader should be able to:

1   Have an insight into the future of paramedic research

2   Recognise the challenges faced for the future of paramedic research

3   Have an understanding of the political influences on paramedic research

4   Identify research topics in paramedic practice

Keywords
challenges
paramedic research
political influences

Introduction

The reader of this book should now have a sound level of understanding of research and its relevance to paramedic practice. We have noted that understanding research and being able to critique research is not merely an academic exercise that you do in college but rather is an essential element of paramedic practice. The future for the paramedic profession as outlined by the College of Paramedics (CoP) (2008) envisages a career structure that embraces research as a key element of the progress from paramedic student through to consultant paramedic. In this final chapter we will draw on aspects discussed in the book and offers suggestions for the development of paramedic research.

Considering your practice

We have drawn a distinction between doers and users of research and have noted that the basic level of paramedic practice requires the ability to read, discuss and draw on research findings. However, as discussed in Chapter 2 we can develop thinking skills to develop and enhance our practice without needing to go on a university course. Undertaking a paramedic preparation programme, at entry to the profession level or at specialist or advanced levels, will provide you with essential knowledge to pass the course. Learning theory (or propositional learning) is, though, only part of the learning that paramedics experience as they also learn by doing (or experiential learning) and working alongside colleagues with other knowledge gained by their own studies and experience. The paramedic is also required to be a critical thinker and to seek answers to questions that arise from practice: to maintain an inquiring and questioning approach to practice. So to develop practice knowledge the practitioner can reflect during and upon clinical situations and so put into an articulated form the tacit knowledge used and from this a theory of practice can develop that can be tested within a research project. To illustrate this point we are going to give you two examples of research studies that arose from practice and were stimulated by the researchers asking 'why?'.

The first example (see Box 11.1) relates to a questioning of accepted practice guidelines whilst applying knowledge from personal experience and a sound understanding of anatomy, physiology, pathophysiology and pharmacology. Coupled with this knowledge base the question reflects the paramedic's desire to do what is best for the patient.

Box 11.1 Use of glucose to treat hypoglycaemia

A paramedic noted that when treating hypoglycaemia in pregnant patients or children a 10% presentation of dextrose was prescribed by JRCLAC guidelines whereas other hypoglycaemic patients were routinely given 50% dextrose.

Pregnant patients and children appeared to recover as well as those given 50%. This question was asked by a practice colleague:

If we can use 10% dextrose for pregnant females, why can't we use it for all adults?

This question leads to a randomised controlled trial (See Box 11.2) and to findings that can improve patient outcomes.

Box 11.2 Setting up the study

Moore and Woollard (2005) 10% or 50% dextrose in the treatment of hypoglycaemia out of hospital? A randomised controlled trial.

A randomised controlled trial was set up aimed to determine whether 10% dextrose is as safe and effective as 50% dextrose when treating hypoglycaemia out-of-hospital. 10% dextrose proved as effective as 50% in the out-of hospital treatment of hypoglycaemia. It is administered in lower doses than a 50% presentation, which results in more acceptable post-treatment blood glucose levels.

To answer this research question a quantitative approach was needed as the findings had to be measurable and have statistical significance so as to answer the research question: 'Did the intervention (the independent variable) make a difference to the outcome (the dependent variable)?' What then if the question had asked instead: 'What are the experiences of carers who have witnessed a hypo-glycaemic episode?' The only way to get that information would be to ask carers who have experiences of the person they care for becoming hypoglycaemic and so a qualitative approach would be required. Both approaches and those research studies that have elements of both (mixed methods) have their place: the method chosen must be suitable to answer the question asked. Currently however the majority of paramedic research is the quantitative type and the development of paramedic research using qualitative methodologies, such as ethnography, will have the potential to further develop paramedic practice (see Box 11.3).

Box 11.3 A qualitative study related to acute medical care

Griffiths (2011) A community of practice: the nurses' role on a medical assessment unit.

An ethnographic approach was used. Data were collected using participant obser-vation, interviewing, and scrutiny of documents. Twenty participants were interviewed including paramedics, doctors, nurses and patients.

Findings indicated that the extreme pressure on beds was a key driver to the organisation of care and all staff were time pressured and experienced workplace stress but friendly and autonomous working patterns mitigated the affects of this stress. One finding related to the lack of attention that the receiving nurse paid to the paramedic's transfer report. This is an area that is suitable for further research and investigation.

Example two relates to a study that came about because Griffiths asked of herself 'How do medical assessment units (MAU) work?' When turning to the literature there was very limited information so Griffiths undertook an ethnography of one MAU for her doctoral study to answer her own question.

This study remains one of the few studies that have considered how MAUs work, despite their presence (or similar) in most district general hospitals in the UK.

What to research?

Students looking to select a research topic for Master's dissertation or doctoral thesis can often identify an issue from their own practice or alternatively by reading paramedic literature can find topic areas that are suitable to be researched. So by reading research papers we can often identify areas of future research that have been raised by the original study. It is difficult to be successful in gaining funding to undertake research; as a small part player in a bigger project is how most researchers begin their careers. Increasingly, funders of research demand that practitioners and service users are involved in the design and conduct of funded studies. This may lead to you being asked to join a large research project to contribute your clinical expertise: this again is a wonderful opportunity to gain research experience in a nurturing and well-supported environment.

Challenges of paramedic research and practice

There are many challenges for the development of healthcare research; this in-cludes paramedic practice. As a registrant of the Health Professions Council you are required to keep your professional knowledge and skills up to date (HPC 2008). Being involved in a research study will help you to enhance your professional prac-tice. One of the challenges of undertaking research however is one of resources. The time and cost to carry out a research study should not be underestimated. Even a small scale study needs employer support ideally, even if that is only to give the researcher some time release from practice. As more and more healthcare professions endeavour to develop their practice through research the competition to obtain funding is becoming greater. It is therefore even more difficult for the novice researcher to find funding for their proposed study, but you may start small in your area of interest and this may lead to greater involvement. Disseminating your work, either from educational programmes or workplace led initiatives, is a very good way to get yourself noticed and many researchers have been invited to join funded projects due to a poster presentation, a publication in a professional journal or a workplace presentation being noticed by research leaders.

Political influences on paramedic research and practice

The world of paramedic science has evolved rapidly over recent years and this growth continues. The challenges of paramedic practice are being led increasingly by political drivers, for example the unscheduled care agenda. The political agenda influences the allocation of funding for those research studies that are seen as a priority. The challenge for the paramedic profession is to compete for this limited funding often in completion with other powerful professions. Also, the paramedic profession itself must influence the political agenda so that what they see as priority areas are researched.

Developing professional knowledge

Professional knowledge is developed on both a micro and macro level: the develop-ment of professional knowledge happens at an individual level and at a professional level. The challenge for the paramedic profession is to develop a unique body of paramedic knowledge to underpin paramedic practice and education. The risk is that other healthcare professions may dominate this development. However, it is recognised that all professions at some point influence one another due to the nature of healthcare, which is rarely delivered by one professional group only.

Influencing your practice through research

All healthcare practice should be evidence based but you do not have to be carrying out research yourself to influence practice. There are many other ways to influence and improve your practice as discussed throughout this book. Jasper et al. (2010) argue that critically reflecting can make an important contribution to the evidence base of health disciplines. Critical reflection gives you a clear structure through which you can question and evaluate your practice. The process of reflection can also help you build upon and expand your existing knowledge base. Reflection can also be part of action research. Action research is different to traditional research and aims to share knowledge and the learning that took place to create that knowledge (McNiff and Whitehead 2009).

Small scale evaluation can also be used to evaluate and influence your practice. Evaluation allows healthcare professionals to make improvements and inform decisions about whether a treatment or process should continue (Brophy et al. 2008). Evaluation of practice incorporates the skills discussed within this book. You should be able to reflect on practice and search and critique the literature as well as learning from your evaluation. When searching literature you should include up-to-date evidence based guidelines from reputable sources as previously discussed. An outcome of your reflection or evaluation of practice should include implementing your findings and considering change in practice where it is necessary.

Personal knowledge

Whilst you are developing your practice through research you will be developing your own personal knowledge. You do not have to be enrolled on an academic programme to do this although it does help to have support. You may attend individual study days or conferences to get ideas to improve your practice. Attending such days gives you the opportunity to network and share ideas. You may set up a journal club where you and your colleagues take turns to present critically appraised research papers. You are required by the HPC to keep a portfolio of your continuing professional development and you can take the opportunity to include these activities in your portfolio. As part of your employment your development will be reviewed mostly now within a 'professional development plan' (PDP). Your PDP should be incorporated into your portfolio demonstrating how you are developing your own professional practice and influencing paramedic practice.

Conclusion

The future of paramedic research relies on both the individual paramedic, and the profession as a whole, grabbing and making opportunities to expand its clinical evidence base. It is evident that paramedic practice can only be developed with the support of reflection, evaluation and research, both small and large scale. The development and expansion of paramedic knowledge can and must be taken forward by the paramedic profession and should not rely on, or be overly influenced by, other healthcare professionals. With the move of paramedic education into higher education paramedics' research skills will be developed and enhanced with the support of academics. It is imperative that paramedics take ownership of their own development and that of their profession so as to build upon the knowledge base of paramedic science and truly move to autonomous professional paramedic practice.

References

Brophy, S., Snooks, H. and Griffiths, L. (2008) *Small-Scale Evaluation in Health: A Practical Guide*. London: Sage.

College of Paramedics. British Paramedic Association (2008) *Paramedic Curriculum Guidance and Competence Framework* (2nd edn). Derby: College of Paramedics.

Griffiths, P. (2011) A community of practice: the nurses' role on a medical assessment unit. *Journal of Clinical Nursing* 20(1–2): 247–254.

Health Professions Council (2008) *Standards of Conducts, Performance and Ethics*. London: HPA.

Jasper, M., Rolfe, G. and Freshwater, D. (2010) *Critical Reflection in Practice: Generating Knowledge for Care* (2nd edn). Basingstoke: Palgrave Macmillan.

McNiff, J. and Whitehead, J. (2009) *Doing and Writing Action Research*. London: Sage.

Moore, C. and Woollard, M. (2005) 10% or 50% dextrose in the treatment of hypoglycaemia out of hospital? A randomised controlled trial. *Emergency Medicine Journal* 22: 512–515.

Further reading

Jasper, M. (2006) *Professional Development, Reflection and Decision-making*. Oxford: Blackwell Publishing.

Koch, T. and Kralik, D. (2006) *Participatory Action Research in Health Care*. Oxford: Blackwell Publishing.

Glossary

Audit trail   evidence provided in a qualitative research report, often in the form of excerpts from the researcher's reflexive journal, that the methodology has been adhered to in a rigorous manner

Case study   a detailed analysis of a single case where the term case represents a location, institution, community or other group

Categorical data   data with discrete values e.g. male, female

Causality   the relationship between the action of one variable that causes an effect on another

Central tendency   a set of scores based around the centre of the score distribution represented by the mean, mode and median

Chi-square   a non-parametrical statistical test used to explore the statistical relationship between two categorical variables

Cluster random sampling   a sampling strategy that involves organising the study population into clusters or groups of similar entities before sub-sampling of the smaller groups

Cohort studies   a study following a cohort (group) of people to determine whether a supposed outcome occurs

Confidence interval   a range of values within which the true value is thought to lie

Confounding factors   a variable, other than the independent variable that may affect a dependent variable

Construct validity   the extent to which a questionnaire reveals data that confirm existing statistical relationships (also known as measurement validity)

Constructionism   the epistemological theory that our access to reality is always mediated through a social or psychological lens. In simple terms, what we see is what we have been taught or conditioned to see rather than what is really there

Continuous data   data measured along a continuum e.g. weight

Control group   the participants in experimental research who do not receive the experimental treatment or intervention. An alternative treatment or placebo may be administered instead

Convenience sampling   selection of people who have information on the topic being studied who can be accessed conveniently to participate in a study

Correlational research   a non-experimental research design in which relationships between variables are explored without any intervention from the researcher

Criterion-related validity   how well a new data collection instrument compares with tried and tested measures

Critical realism   a 'softer' form of constructionism which recognises the existence of an objective reality but questions our ability to perceive it with any degree of certainty

Cronbach's alpha   a reliability index that measures the consistency of the questions within a scale

Data saturation   the point in a qualitative research study at which no new findings are being produced. Data saturation is often used to determine the sample size

Dependant variable   the variable thought to be influenced by or depend on another

Descriptive statistics   statistics used to summarise and present data, usually presented as frequencies or percentages

Double blind studies   an experimental study in which both researcher and subject are unaware of who has been allocated to the control and experimental groups

Ecological validity   the extent to which the findings of a study are applicable to the participants' natural social settings

Epistemology   the philosophical study of the nature, constitution and origins of knowledge

Evidence based practice   practice based on research, professional and patient experience

External reliability   consistency when questionnaires are administered at different times within the same population, also known as stability

External validity   the degree to which the behaviour and opinions of the sample population are representative of the wider population

Experimental research   a methodology in which the researcher attempts to control and/or manipulate all the relevant variables in order to take measurements that are not distorted by extraneous factors

Expert practice   expert practice is usually defined in healthcare settings as practice based predominantly on the accumulated experience of the practitioner rather than simply on the application of findings from research

Fisher's exact tests   a method of testing the significance of the relationship between categorical variables when the sample size is small

Generalisable   research findings are said to be generalisable when they can be applied to a larger group than that from which they were generated. Qualitative and quantitative researchers usually have different approaches to ensuring generalisability

Hypothesis   a prediction that a relationship between variables will be established

Hypothetico-deductivism   an alternative to inductivism in which the aim is to attempt to disprove a research hypothesis. Continued failure to disprove a hypothesis allows us to have a degree of confidence in its truthfulness or validity

Independent variable   the variable that is thought to influence or manipulate the dependent variable

Inferential statistics   statistics that allow inferences to be made from the sample population that can be applied to the general population

Interrator reliability   the level of agreement among two or more independent observers participating in an observation simultaneously

Internal validity   the degree to which cause and effect can be demonstrated

Internal reliability   (or consistency) is a measure of the extent to which instruments within a scale measure the construct being studied

Interval measurement   rank ordering of data where a regular interval is apparent between the categories but no absolute zero is present

Intervention group   the participants in experimental research who receive the experimental treatment or intervention (also known as the experimental group)

Kruskal-Wallis test   a non-parametric test designed to test the difference between the ranked scores of three or more independent groups

Likert scales   a scale utilising predetermined scores in which participants indicate their level of agreement (or disagreement)

Mann-Whitney *U* test   a non-parametric test designed to test the difference between the ranked scores of two independent groups

Mean   a measure of central tendency described as the sum of all values divided by the number of values in your dataset

Median   a measure of central tendency described as the value above and below which an equal number of cases occur

Methods   the data collection tools employed in a research study. For example, a 'tick-box' questionnaire is a quantitative research method and an interview is a qualitative method

Methodology   the overarching philosophical framework that directs the conduct of the study. For example, a survey is a quantitative methodology and a phenomenological study is a qualitative methodology

Mixed-methods research   combines both quantitative and qualitative approaches to collect and analyse data

Mode   a measure of central tendency described as the most frequently occurring value in a distribution of scores

Naturalistic research   unlike experimental research, naturalistic approaches attempt to gather data 'in the field' without interfering with or manipulating the sources of the data

Negative skew   an asymmetrical distribution of values where the long tail of the graph is directed in a negative direction indicating that the majority of values are clustered at the high end of the distribution

Nominal measurement   the lowest form of measurement and relates to assignment into categories that can be named and assigned a numerical code (e.g. paramedic category 1 and emergency medical technician, category 2)

Non-experimental   a study in which the independent variables are not manipulated

Non-probability sampling   the selection of participants with no attempt at randomisation

Null hypothesis   the prediction that no relationship between variables will be established

Ontology   the philosophical study of the nature and constitution of reality

Ordinal measurement   a level of measurement that allows sorting of data based on a ranking system where order is apparent between each category but not quantifiable (e.g. fair, category 1; good, category 2; excellent, category 3)

Paradigm   a set of assumptions about the nature of knowledge shared by members of a particular research community

Placebo   an inactive substance often given to the control group in an experimental study

Practitioner research   research conducted by practitioners, usually focussing on their own practice, their own clinical area, or the practice of their immediate colleagues. Practitioner research is therefore a form of insider research

Pretest-posttest design   a research design in which data are collected before (pretest) and after (posttest) an intervention

Positive skew   an asymmetrical distribution of values where the long tail of the graph is directed in a positive direction indicating that the majority of values are clustered at the low end of the distribution

Probability sampling   random selection of participants from a population by utilising a sampling frame of list of potential participants

Propositional knowledge   knowledge that can be expressed in terms of formal propositions that results from or can be subject to scientific testing

Prospective studies   a study in which current phenomena are explored by moving forward in time to collect data

Purposive sampling   selection of research participants based on the researcher's judgement on their suitability for inclusion

Qualitative   includes all studies that collect data in formats other than numbers. However, it is also used in a more philosophical sense to describe studies that do not subscribe to the 'hard science' research paradigm

Quantitative   includes all studies that collect data in the form of numbers. However, it is also used in a more philosophical sense to describe studies that subscribe to the scientific research paradigm

Quasi-experiments   experimental research where randomisation is not possible

Quota sampling   a method of sampling in which certain characteristics within a sample are deliberately sought e.g. ethnicity or gender

Randomised controlled trial   experimental research incorporating randomisation of a sample into experimental and control groups

Random sampling   a sampling technique that ensures that each member of a population has an equal chance of inclusion

Randomisation   the random allocation of subjects into groups

Range   a measure of central tendency described as the highest minus the lowest score in a dataset

Ratio measurement   rank ordering of data where an absolute zero is present

Realism   the philosophical theory that the world can be perceived directly and more or less accurately through our senses

Reflection in action   a term coined by Donald Schön to describe a process of thinking and reflecting whilst in the midst of practice

Reflection on action   a term coined by Donald Schön to describe a process of thinking and reflecting away from and after practice has taken place

Reflexivity   an awareness that the social researcher cannot achieve an entirely objective position when conducting a study of the social world

Reliability a term used mainly by quantitative researchers to describe the accuracy of their data collection tools both over time and between different researchers

Reliability coefficient a quantitative measure of the degree of reliability

Retrospective study a study in which information from the past is used to explain current events

Sample a representative sub-set of a population

Significance testing a method by which researchers determine whether a relationship between variables could have occurred by chance

Single blind study an experimental study in which the researcher is unaware of who has been allocated to the control or experimental group

Snowball sampling a form of convenience sampling where participants recommend others that they think will be suitable participants

Stratified random sampling a form of sampling that involves organising the target population into strata or divisions according to predetermined characteristics before implementing random sampling

Survey a method of obtaining data from a sample population through direct questioning

Tacit knowledge knowledge that cannot easily be expressed in words, for example, the knowledge required to ride a bicycle. Tacit knowledge can be contrasted with propositional knowledge

Test-retest reliability a measure of the stability of an instrument involving comparing the scores achieved on repeated administrations

Variable something that varies

Validity (quantitative) the extent to which a data collection instrument measures what it purports to measure

Validity (qualitative) a term used mainly by qualitative researchers to describe the 'truth value' i.e. how accurately findings represent the social phenomena studied

Index